FROM LIVING HELL TO LIVING WELL

Reclaim Your Health & Happiness
With the Power of a Holistic Approach

HEIDI & STEVE JENNINGS

NOTE FROM THE AUTHORS

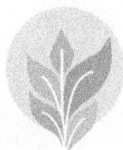

The information contained in this book is based on our experience and success within our coaching practice. We do not give advice about medication and any decisions regarding these should be discussed with your doctor.

Real names have been used for our case studies in Chapter 11 and for all testimonials. Where there are references to other clients within the book, names have been changed to protect their privacy.

TESTIMONIALS

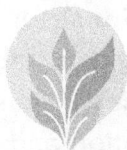

"For seven years, I suffered mostly from migraines; the last one I had caused me to sleep for 24 hours. I used a $700 physio programme that gave me few results and powerful medications from doctors with no resolve. Steve and Heidi's approach was completely natural, alternative and holistic. Since starting the plan, I have not had one migraine and I haven't needed my medications. The words 'thank you' are not enough!"

Alice, 40s

"The programme is great for my lifestyle. I know I can have a night or two off each week, allow my weight to come up a little over the weekend, then easily drop the weight over the week. I'm down 10kg already in just a couple of months. The food is easy, I sleep better than ever, my stress is far more manageable and I'm not missing out on social events. This programme is so easy once you know how the system works."

Nigel, 50s

"I was exercising HARD four to five times per week and couldn't lose weight. Once I got on Steve and Heidi's programme, they told me to stop exercising. I was sceptical at first but they were right! I dropped 7kg in just 42 days and I only walked once. I'm at my lightest weight in 25 years!"

Shar, 50s

"I had been struggling with several health issues for many years, including fibromyalgia, Irritable Bowel Syndrome (IBS), costochondritis, daily anxiety, sinus problems, gut problems such as bloating, constipation and diarrhoea, joint pain and inflammation, excess weight, and an overall feeling of being very unwell. After just six weeks on the programme, my irritable bowel symptoms, indigestion and irregular bowel patterns were gone. The glands around my neck and under my arms reduced to the point I can no longer feel them. I started sleeping better and stopped taking anti-histamine medication because my sinuses have settled down. My anxiety has lessened a lot and I feel like I'm on a much more even keel now. This programme has been the best thing I've ever done for my health and I'm so pleased with how far I've come."

Tania, 40s

"Before starting Steve and Heidi's programme, I was dealing with a whole raft of health issues. Some stressful life events had led me down the path of over-eating, not sleeping well, dealing with chronic anxiety and I was also suffering from daily headaches and occasional severe migraines. I had very little energy and was struggling in general with my health. Within the first few weeks my migraines disappeared, I had much more energy, and my anxiety significantly reduced. The meals were easy and tasty and by the end of two weeks I had lost 4kg! I would highly recommend this programme to anyone needing to take control of their physical and mental health."

Lauren, 30s

"I had constant hot flushes during the night and spent about $5,000 on menopause treatments that didn't work. I got used to hearing the same information over and over again from each professional I spoke to. I am amazed at how easy Steve and Heidi's plan is to follow. I lost 5kg in two weeks and I exercised less than ever. My hot flushes at night have reduced to one or two per night after just six weeks."

Jill, 50s

First published by Ultimate World Publishing 2021
Copyright © 2021 Heidi & Steve Jennings

ISBN

Paperback: 978-1-922597-99-1
Ebook: 978-1-922714-00-8

Cover design: Ultimate World Publishing
Layout and typesetting: Ultimate World Publishing
Editor: Alex Floyd-Douglass

ULTIMATE WORLD
—— PUBLISHING ——

Ultimate World Publishing
Diamond Creek,
Victoria Australia 3089
www.writeabook.com.au

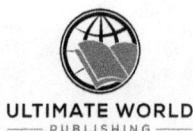

For Bonnie and Arie,

True happiness comes from finding what lights you up, then pursuing it with courage and faith. And from eating your vegetables.

All our love always,
Mum and Dad

CONTENTS

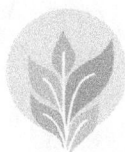

PREFACE

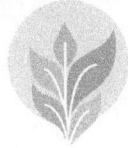

We talked about writing a book for a long time because we know our message is life-changing and needs to be shared far and wide. Building a business over the best part of 20 years brings with it plenty of sweat and sleepless nights, but also a wealth of priceless knowledge and experience. Eventually, it came to fruition when circumstances allowed for the time and energy to make it happen.

We are immensely proud of this book because it represents not only our holistic health coaching business but the strength of our partnership as a couple after the trials we survived. We are grateful for every life experience – whether high or low and both individually and together – because each one has brought us to where we are today, doing a job we love and living a life we could only dream of.

Our mission is to share our message with and impact 500,000 people around the world. Ultimately though, we want to help those who need it the most, by leading the way and showing them how to become the vital and vibrant beings they were born to be.

"He who has health, has hope;
and he who has hope, has everything."

(Thomas Carlyle)

IT'S TIME TO LEAVE YOUR LIVING HELL

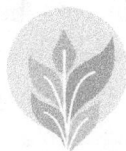

Dealing with pain, chronic illness or a general feeling of mediocrity is nobody's idea of fun – and it's certainly no way to live. If you've picked up this book because you're stuck in your own version of hell, whether it's discomfort or dissatisfaction, if something isn't feeling quite right, or you just know you're not at your best, this is an exciting time for you.

The information we are about to share has already changed the lives of thousands of people and will continue to do so well into the future. Who are we to be so confident you ask? Well, you better keep reading!

Firstly though, let's back up a step. The next time you go to work or walk down the street, take a look at the people around you. Are they happy, smiling and bursting with positivity? Or are they tired, sluggish and stressed?

Our bet is that for every individual in the first category, there are 10 in the second.

Life in the 21st century has led to a population of individuals who for the most part plod through their days, months and years in so-so shape. They do what needs to be done to achieve the things they think they should.

By 40, there's some middle-age spread and a few aches and pains going on, but that's a normal part of the ageing process, right? By 50, there's a few more niggles, maybe an autoimmune condition and a sense that life isn't working out quite as planned. 65 comes along and now it's all about pill popping to keep the blood pressure and cholesterol in check along with a looming fear that the golden years aren't looking too rosy.

Because we see so many people around us who are sick and overwhelmed, we begin to think it's normal. Common, yes. Normal, definitely not. Each of us was born into a body whose most primal desire is to thrive. Over a lifetime, we accumulate a pile of stressors and traumas that one by one can kill that primal urge – if we allow them.

Perhaps you are reading these words and feeling uncomfortable with how they resonate with you. Perhaps you are struggling with any manner of health conditions that your doctor has written off as 'incurable' or require a lifetime of medication. Or perhaps you are feeling okay right now, but you know some of your less-than-great habits could use a tweak. Only you know what's really going on for you – and what needs to change.

Life isn't always easy, but it's certainly a lot worse when you don't have good health on your side.

We know this first-hand, because we've been there. We also know that a glorious sense of wellness – where you have energy to burn and a smile on your dial to light up the room – is absolutely within your reach and it's there for the taking, no matter how miserable you might be feeling right now. The difference between those who have this sublime state of health and those who don't is all about *knowing how to get it*.

We know you might be struggling right now. Chronic pain, depression, anxiety, stubborn body fat, menopause symptoms, sleep issues, autoimmune dysfunction... Whatever it is that is bringing you down, we hear you. And we are here for you. We also know how to help you restore your sparkle, your sense of humour and love of life. And we're going to share it with you right here and now.

This book is for you if you're feeling stuck, confused or frustrated, with no idea where to turn next.

It's for you if your gut is telling you there's more to life than the daily grind with a body that refuses to cooperate.

It's for you if you are ready to embrace the exhilarating opportunity of grasping the steering wheel and living life on your terms.

Most of the information in the following chapters is not going to be anything you hear inside your doctor's office. That's because we take a holistic approach, where we heal the body from the inside out by getting to the root cause of the problem. We're not interested in medicating you up to the eyeballs to mask symptoms and pretend they're not really there. We're interested in your ability to throw your medication in the bin, restore the bright whites of your eyeballs and ultimately, start living.

We know you're ready, so what are you waiting for?

Let's go!

CHAPTER ONE

ROCK BOTTOM – HEIDI'S STORY

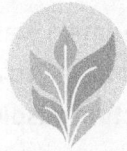

"*Do you really think I can get better?*" I asked my husband Steve for the umpteenth time, as I lay in bed clutching his hand, skin burning, sweat dripping, thoughts blurred from lack of sleep.

"*Yes, you can,*" he said, "*And when we figure out what's going on, we're going to be able to help a lot of people.*"

At that point, I didn't care about anything except escaping the nightmare I was in. Fear and exhaustion were steering the ship and I was struggling to see a way out.

Chronic illness was my undoing. It was also my greatest blessing. Let me explain.

7

Early 2015

After outgrowing our small abode, Steve and I, along with our two young children, built a beautiful new home in a rural community, a 15-minute drive from the city. Steve was running our fitness business, I was a full-time mum, our children were still pre-schoolers and we were happy. Life was good.

Everything changed for me 18 months later, as a range of curious physical symptoms started to appear, the first of which was a rash that spread across my neck, chest and torso.

With a lifelong history of eczema, I was used to red and itchy skin, but this was different. I had learned to control the eczema through my diet and I had an instinctual suspicion these symptoms were related to something in our immediate environment.

My efforts to figure out the cause were extensive but yielded nothing and I was getting nowhere, fast.

January 2017

One morning as I went to get out of bed, my whole world tipped upside down. I had to put my hand on the wall to steady myself as the most horrendous spinning sensation overtook me. I collapsed back onto the bed, knowing immediately it was vertigo.

Each time I turned my head, the spinning would return so intensely that I felt sure I would vomit. I attempted to get in the shower but couldn't balance. I was scared; what on earth was going on?

It took two trips to two different doctors to confirm my original self-diagnosis of vertigo.

Over the next few days, episodes of repetitive intense spinning left me housebound and terrified. I lost my confidence to go out in public or transport my kids in the car. I stopped exercising. I had no idea why I was so unwell and no clue how to fix it. The doctor was able to give me a helpful manoeuvre to restore balance during an episode, but it didn't prevent the vertigo from returning over and over again.

Very soon after the onset of vertigo, another symptom in the form of eye floaters joined the party. Eye surgery in my left eye a few years prior had resulted in some floating debris, but for the most part, they didn't bother me.

Suddenly, I had multiple insect-shaped floaters obstructing my line of vision and the timing was too coincidental to ignore.

My attempts to figure out what was making me sick were ongoing over a period of months and eventually, a phone call to the local council confirmed the land directly opposite us was contaminated with arsenic. Because the land was undergoing development, by law the pockets of contamination had to be removed.

I have a vivid memory of the windy summer and layers of dust that infiltrated our house that year and shudder with horror. At the time though, we were clueless to the fact we were breathing in arsenic.

After much heartache, we had to acknowledge that our home was making me sick and we needed to move away from the area. I thought things were pretty bad at this point and had no idea that 'bad' was about to turn into 'nightmare.'

9

Before learning how food sensitivities were linked to eczema, I had used steroid creams to combat the odd patch that would pop up from time to time. Several years earlier, I had learned about a 'rebound effect' that can happen when stopping steroid use.

The skin goes into a form of shock and needs to learn to function normally again without steroids. It can lead to cycles of flaring (redness) and flaking until correct skin function is restored. In hindsight, I had already been through a mild case of that years before when I ceased using steroids and started to eliminate problematic foods.

Toxic Heavy Metal Poisoning

By April 2017, that was a distant memory and I was in a bad way. Against my better judgement, I decided to use a steroid cream to help with the rash that by now was starting to crack and was unbearably itchy. I went to my doctor to ask for hydrocortisone (the mildest steroid cream) and he happily obliged.

The next few weeks passed in a blur as we moved back to the city and hair testing confirmed I had toxic heavy metal poisoning. I was using the steroid cream sparingly, but I noticed the rash was worsening and spreading further down my body. I realised I was in the beginning stages of the 'rebound effect.'

Topical Steroid Withdrawal

After just nine weeks of steroid cream use, I was a mess. My eyelids had become puffy and swollen and the skin had started to flake. My cheeks and upper lip were red and patchy. Doctor Google had told me all about Topical Steroid Withdrawal (TSW) and I was at the very beginning of the process. I remember looking in the mirror and praying that I would be let off lightly.

I thought just nine weeks of use might spare me the horror of what I had seen on those wretched faces of the people on Google. I was wrong.

Within three days, I was sobbing uncontrollably on the couch. A bone-deep itch had kicked in and I had clawed my face to shreds. While I silently hoped the symptoms would pass quickly, instinctively I knew things weren't good and I was in for a tough time.

June rolled into July, August and beyond – and my skin was worsening every day. My entire neck and chest were covered in a rash. My face was bright red and was moving through cycles of flaring, flaking and oozing. My eyes were swollen and puffy. My inner elbows, lower abdomen and the backs of my knees erupted in severe cracking and bleeding. The rash spread from my shoulders down to my elbows. My arms were heavily bandaged because they were mutilated by my fingernails and bleeding badly.

I stopped using our upstairs shower because I couldn't stand looking at myself in the mirror. I couldn't sleep at night because the itch was too severe. I would purposely scratch until I bled because the pain was preferable to the itch. My skin started flaking multiple times a day. My ear lobes were scabbed and bleeding. I had wounds all over my scalp where I had scratched too hard. I needed band aids and bandages on my face to mop up the ooze.

Each time I gently removed a band aid, a layer of skin would come with it, leaving more open wounds. I developed night sweats and would wake up with soaking wet sheets, multiple times every single night. Steve slept in another bed for months on end because he still had to go to work each day and my itching kept him awake.

I spent entire nights in tears because I was so exhausted and sleep was nowhere to be found. I would eventually drift off to sleep at around 5am and would be in no state to get up at 7am to get the kids off to school. Most mornings, I had to kiss them goodbye from my bed, using all my strength not to cry buckets of guilty tears.

Physically, I looked like I had been burned and mentally I wasn't doing much better. Over a period of months, there were endless rounds of tears, swearing and feelings of disbelief that this was my reality.

I was deeply unhappy and scared and had no idea how long I would be in this hell; TSW has no definitive end date.

Meanwhile, Steve was responsible for keeping our business and family afloat. He spent hours running his fingers up and down my arms and back to soothe the itch, telling me he loved me no matter what. The stress on him was immense but he shouldered all of it, while constantly reassuring me that I needed to have faith and that I would be well again.

"There is going to be a huge lesson in all of this," he would say, *"We just don't know what it is yet."*

I held on to that for dear life and will never forget the pillar of strength he was for me at that time. He did everything he could to ease my burden of stress so I could focus on rest and recovery.

Not many people around me understood what was going on because TSW is not a well-known condition. This was an incredibly lonely period in my life where I felt abandoned by certain friends and family who didn't know how to handle illness, ignored it completely or simply couldn't be bothered with it all. It taught me a lot about who my true supporters are and was a stark lesson in self-reliance.

July 2018

After a full year of TSW symptoms, I developed a bacterial infection on my face from the open wounds. Up until this point, I had resisted going to the doctor because I knew the medical community does not acknowledge TSW. It is an absolute tragedy that doctors do not recognise the devastating effects of topical steroids. They continue to dish them out like candy on a global scale, meanwhile overlooking the fact that millions of people are suffering unnecessarily.

I knew I needed antibiotics to clear up the infection though, so going to the doctor was essential. My face was not only bright red, flaking and oozing, it was now covered in scabs and my left eye was swollen shut. I will never forget the stares I got as I walked into that waiting room.

Sure enough, my doctor disputed my claims of TSW and I walked out of her office feeling utterly lost and alone. I cried all the way home in the car and I remember the feeling of total despair in the pit of my stomach. I was still getting regular bouts of vertigo and eye floaters, I was physically disfigured with a bacterial infection to boot and I had no support from my doctor.

That was the absolute lowest point in my life.

It was also the most crucial turning point, because it was right then and there, during the soul-destroying drive home, that I had

13

my epiphany moment – without which I would not be where I am today as a coach and this book would never have been written.

Healing

Rock bottom takes you to a deeply lonely place where it's natural to become paralysed by the mind.

Certainly, at my rock bottom, while my mother was driving me home from the doctor, all I could feel was hopelessness and fear. It was also the moment I realised I was completely alone in my fight to recover.

My doctor wouldn't help me. My friends and family couldn't help me. It was just me, on my own, desperately needing to figure out a way to climb out of the pit. It was so stark a realisation that I call it my epiphany; a lightbulb moment that happened in my darkest hour.

I have to be honest and reveal that I had a few moments over those long months and years where I didn't want to keep living. At my absolute lowest point, I silently begged to die in my sleep. I didn't feel strong enough to cope with what was happening to my body and mind and I felt myself slipping into a deep hole. I didn't believe I was capable of taking my own life, but I definitely had times when I wanted it to be taken from me. It's not something I am proud of but it was my reality at the time and I now realise it was a very natural result of declining physical and mental health.

At this point, I knew I had two options. I could continue to wallow in the despair and misery, or I could fight with all my might. I knew which one I would choose, because I was damned if I was giving in. Ultimately, I just wanted to be well again and live a full and happy life.

I became determined to find a way out.

I started devouring any information I could find on healing; anything that could give me a smidgen of hope. Because I already understood deeply how food affected my body, this became an area I focused on. I had already removed some 'trouble-makers' from my diet, but I realised I needed to dig deeper and take things to a new level.

I delved heavily into the plant-based diet and the more I researched about this way of life, the more it made sense to me. Food was going to be my medicine!

Around this time, the idea of cooking meat was making me feel ill and I told Steve I didn't want to cook it anymore. Because I was so sick, he was very understanding and wanted to support me in whatever I needed to do to get better. To this day, the smell of raw meat makes me want to hurl. Experimenting with new foods and recipes was my beacon of light in a very dark time and I couldn't believe the beautiful meals with so much rich flavour that I was able to create.

The healing process was frustratingly slow and was definitely not linear. Positive changes started to occur at the 18 month mark, but I continued to go through cyclical patterns of recurring symptoms with my skin. I learned a lot about the need for patience while healing the body and I developed a deep trust in my body that it was incredibly intelligent and knew exactly what it was doing. This helped immensely during the cycles of recurring symptoms, where I was able to reassure myself that the body had to go through the cycle to get to the next phase of healing.

Meanwhile, my vertigo and eye floaters were starting to subside and I knew without a shadow of a doubt that my diet of beautiful, whole, nutrient-dense foods were helping me heal.

Mid 2019

Two years after the start of my symptoms, I had come a long way. There were still ups and downs and Steve would continue to remind me that we were in the middle of a huge lesson, even though we had no clarity around what it was. Because I was in much better shape physically and mentally, I was able to appreciate that he was absolutely right and I started thinking hard about what those lessons might be.

I also began to realise that between Steve and I, we had collected a vast amount of valuable knowledge and resources, as we were both constantly seeking out new information, researching alternative medicine, trying new foods and healing techniques and putting all the puzzle pieces together. Steve had recently shifted direction in our business from personal training to finding his niche in health coaching, more accurately reflecting his skills and life experience.

I was delighted for him and was over the moon to be getting better, but the truth was, personally I felt very lost. My confidence had plummeted during those few years because I had spent a lot of time alone and at home. I loved my role as a full-time mum but began to appreciate that my reservoir of inner-strength, experience and knowledge could take me in a powerful new direction.

I realised I had a valuable story to share but didn't have any idea how I could do that.

By now, I was very comfortable with a plant-based diet and I decided to complete a course in plant-based nutrition studies offered through Cornell University in the USA. I knew this would complement my existing life coaching qualification and our health coaching business beautifully. The thought that Steve and I could work together to bring about so many positive changes to other peoples' lives was incredibly exciting and I couldn't wait to get started.

The path from that moment has been absolutely wonderful.

Our respective skills complement each other perfectly and we enjoy spending our time together to formulate life-changing coaching programmes for our clients.

Throughout my health crisis, we spent weeks, months and years doing the rigour and earning our stripes. Steve's earlier words about being able to help many other people have come to fruition in a way we could never have imagined.

As for our big lesson — which was never clear at the time but is crystal clear now — we have come to realise that we could never have developed such outstanding coaching programmes which are utterly transformational for our clients, without going through those years of utter despair.

I am so privileged to be able to share my knowledge and life experience with our clients and now, with you. I am incredibly grateful for what I went through because it brought me here today.

I wouldn't change that for the world.

CHAPTER TWO

IGNITING THE SPARK — STEVE'S STORY

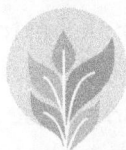

I remember the 10-minute walk home from school, past the state houses that hold stories of their own in a small working-class town. The last few houses before mine have stories of domestic violence, gang parties, drugs and alcohol. State houses that have been passed down within families from one generation to the next.

Then our house; an ex-state house, looked after well. This house has a different story and is the one I'm most familiar with. White weatherboard, three bedrooms, built after the Second World War. The inside is a little weary, but it's humble and hospitable. Beaten into submission at times with teenagers, it still holds its own, perched proudly on the corner of Clive and Beach road.

As I walk across the front lawn, I have a strong sense of anxiety. I'm worried about my mother. She's all I have and she's not very well.

I never had a relationship with my father and my older brothers and sisters have left home. I'm the youngest of five kids.

I'm not sure what mood Mum is going to be in. Sometimes she's in tears, sometimes in pain, sometimes just a little tired, but okay. Mum has Chronic Fatigue Syndrome (CFS). She's bedridden, frequently has physical pain and due to our financial situation and a lack of family support, the stress can be overwhelming.

Being just a child, I am ill-equipped to handle such a situation. Mum can experience bouts of depression and anxiety at times and because she is who I rely on, it's extremely unsettling for me to see my parent falling apart. Some days, she only gets out of bed to use the bathroom. If she works in the garden for a day, she might be exhausted for the next three days or more.

The Journey Begins

For me, my training ground for health coaching started when I was 10 years old. After multiple doctors' visits and no answers, Mum was finally diagnosed with CFS by a specialist. With my mother bed-ridden and exhausted, I started the transition to primary caregiver.

For the next three years, my job involved cooking dinner, cleaning, vegetable gardening, occasional grocery shopping, paying bills and being the shoulder for my mother to cry on. Occasionally during school nights, I would wake up hearing my mother crying because of the physical pain she was in and so I then became the physical therapist, too – stroking her hair to try and ease her pain.

Because Mum couldn't work, we were very poor. On school mufti days, I went to school in my uniform because we didn't have 50 cents in the house for a donation to the school. I just told everyone that I hated mufti day, rather than say we didn't have the money because that was too embarrassing.

My mother was very religious and I was taught all the ins and outs of Catholicism. We had to pray the rosary daily and attend church each week, so I was brought up in a house of faith.

I could not understand why I was born into this situation.

I felt unlucky, lacked confidence and felt very isolated. I had a great burden of loyalty, because when my mother was so unwell and due to some of the religious beliefs I was brought up with, I was told many times, *"You're the only one I can trust."*

My parents had split up before I was born and I never had a connection with my father. I never spent time with him unless I saw him at my grandparents' house for family gatherings, perhaps once or twice per year.

I never felt any support or a sense of leadership from him.

I remember as a seven-year-old, two boys were living two doors down from me and their dad would visit them every now and then and bring them a toy each. I asked the older boy, *"Why does your dad bring you two toys that are exactly the same?"*

He told me that it was so they didn't become jealous of each other and start fighting. I grew quite jealous of these boys and I wondered why my dad didn't visit and bring me toys. And so, I acted out and started stealing toys from them because I was jealous of their relationship with their father.

Eventually, they found out and their mum stepped in and said she'd ring the cops if I kept stealing. And with a vivid seven-year-old imagination I could see myself getting bundled into the back of a police car with handcuffs, being taken to jail, so I promptly gave up on my short-lived thieving career.

By the time I was in college, I felt a huge weight of isolation. I had continuous thoughts like *"No one understands, no one cares, there's no way out, why me, no money, the world is a bad place, there's no light at the end of the tunnel and I'm the only one my mother can trust, so I better behave..."*

My understanding of life at this point was that a noble life is one with a lot of pain and poverty and that's what gets you to Heaven.

As I moved through my teens and into my early twenties, I developed a hatred toward my father that I held onto for a number of years. I had seen him briefly at various family gatherings where he made small talk with a few sentences and that was it.

I had the impression he didn't want to connect with me.

I was waiting for him to invite me to go fishing or come over and stay sometime, but he never did. I felt let down and developed some real anger towards him. He later tried to connect with me at various points between the ages of 15 and 21 but I was bitter and resentful.

I started to avoid my mother's health issues by moving overseas to Australia to earn good money so that I could move ahead and also provide financial assistance to her. This was a time of searching for me, where I wanted to escape poverty and create distance from the burdens at home. It was in Australia that I studied to become a personal trainer using my life savings to fund my tuition.

Sadly, I actually ran out of money when I studied in Sydney so I had to return home.

After I started my own fitness business and at the age of 26, I met Heidi and less than two years later, we were married. A year later, Heidi fell pregnant and we were expecting our beautiful baby girl. I was driven to be a good father and provide my daughter and wife with a stable household.

At about 37 weeks pregnant and on maternity leave, Heidi visited an optometrist because she was having some problems with her eye. This is where my next journey begins.

I remember Heidi ringing me in tears and asking me to come to the eye clinic urgently. The optometrist had found that the retina in her left eye had detached and the right eye was close to detachment, too.

Heidi would have to undergo urgent eye surgery in both eyes at 38 weeks pregnant or she would face permanent blindness. This situation was the first in a chain of health events for Heidi that together, we would encounter over the following eight years.

Two months after the eye surgery, Heidi fell ill with osteomyelitis in her foot – an extremely painful and serious bone infection. Heidi spent two weeks in hospital while I looked after six-week-old Bonnie at home. Heidi would spend the next six weeks in a wheelchair with a new-born baby, still unable to see in her left eye after surgery.

For me personally, this was not a hard time. That was yet to come.

Forgiveness

As I moved into my thirties, I still felt anger, bitterness and hatred towards my father. I had held onto those negative feelings for about 20 years and there was no end in sight. I had been experiencing recurring dreams about him and felt drained. I felt it was my right to be upset and was waiting for an apology.

Eventually, I gave up waiting and came to realise that unless I changed the way I thought about him, I was actually hurting myself and nothing was going to change.

The breakthrough came when I realised I had to reverse all of these feelings by using forgiveness as the solution. I wrote him a letter expressing this forgiveness. By doing so, I had to consciously break the habit of the constant negativity I directed at him.

I expressed forgiveness when we caught up in person and at family gatherings, which eased the tension between us. I also chose to forgive because I didn't want to pass my bitterness onto my kids, affecting their relationship with their grandfather.

I didn't want my children to have to take sides.

The emotional healing that I received from this exercise brought a great sense of relief. The next challenge would be another health issue with Heidi.

A Health Crisis

After our son, Arie, was born in 2013, we decided with a growing family it was time to up-size our house and in 2015, we built a house in the country. We settled into a small, quiet village, Bonnie was about to start school, we were enjoying a nice lifestyle in a brand-new home and our small business was doing well. We were happy.

Little did we know that our happy life was about to be turned upside down.

Heidi has suffered from eczema her entire life; it's her body's way of telling her that something is not right. And her body was about to send us a very important message.

After our first 18 months in the new house, Heidi's skin started to flare up. Her skin was very red, dry and itchy. She had started experiencing vertigo so badly that she couldn't get out of bed and move around or drive. Doctors' tests uncovered nothing abnormal.

This was the beginning of a two-year journey.

Heidi started to become depressed with the way her skin looked because it was all over her face, neck and chest. She often stayed in bed because the vertigo was so debilitating and I frequently found her in tears.

A call to the local council confirmed that the land across the road being developed was previously farm land and was contaminated with arsenic. As the land was being stirred up in the development process, our environment had become very toxic. Heidi's body was very sensitive so she had a harsh reaction, whereas nobody else in the family had any noticeable symptoms.

We moved house and began a recovery phase to remove the heavy metals from her system. It was at this point she had her hair tested and found that her levels of arsenic, mercury and aluminium were off the charts, confirming our suspicion of toxic heavy metal poisoning.

Heidi had started to detox very heavily from some steroid medication she had used to help manage her eczema. She experienced intense itching so bad that her skin bled and she would writhe in tears of agony on the floor.

A painful skin rash had spread across her face, chest and down her arms. She would stay awake all night, leading to complete exhaustion in the morning. She had feelings of intense guilt because she was unable to attend school and pre-school events or get the kids off to school in the morning. She also felt like she was letting me down as a wife.

My job became carer of the kids, caring for Heidi, running the business and running the household duties while Heidi slipped into a depression due to her ongoing severe symptoms. Heidi became so sick that at times she said, *"I don't know if I can carry on. I don't want to live anymore. I don't know if I can get better. I feel like I am a burden on everyone."*

She had become isolated and wouldn't leave the house. We had lost the basics of our relationship; going out for a coffee, socialising as a couple and even being able to sleep in the same bed.

At this point, I was starting to wonder why I had become the carer again. Why was I going through this all over again?

I thought that I had already done my work caring for my mother 25 years ago as a 10 year-old boy. I thought that the hardest part of my life was over. Now I had a sick wife who couldn't leave the house and was very depressed.

26

My Breakthrough

I never had a problem with Heidi being sick. I knew she needed lots of love, compassion and someone she could lean on. My mother-in-law often said to me, *"I don't know how you do it Steve. How do you cope with all of this?"*

And I would reply, *"I've done this all before."*

Heidi would apologise to me for being unwell and I would say, *"Don't worry, I've been through this before."*

And just like that, BANG! After 25 years, I realised the reason I had gone through the journey as a carer for my mother was in preparation to give me the tools and the strength to go through this journey with Heidi.

This was a real epiphany moment.

I now had a reason for that journey as my mother's carer. Now I had a purpose. And now, I had some answers.

The journey that I went through as a carer for my Mum was not a bad thing at all. Yes, it was hard, but it was a necessary experience to provide me with the strength and faith for this journey with Heidi.

Heidi needed someone to lean on and I could be that person.

I fully trusted that Heidi would eventually recover. At her lowest point she would ask me, *"Do you really think I'm going to get better?"*

I would always reply, *"Yes, I've got no doubt you'll get better. And we are going to use this experience to help many people."*

To trust my gut instinct and have faith that everything was going to work out was a real test. There were so many emotions involved, but I kept my emotions out of it so that the kids had some stability at home and so Heidi could lean on me.

After about two years, slowly but surely Heidi started to turn a corner and her skin slowly started to heal. She had now returned to normal function and was back to being herself again.

With all the learning and research we've done over the years, we have been able to develop a safe and natural programme to help our clients take control of their health and start to heal.

Nothing about our journey was easy and it certainly wasn't planned. Those two years were the most difficult of our lives, but would we change anything?

No, because it's brought us to where we are today. We are incredibly grateful for the lessons and opportunities this experience provided us and we are proud of how we've turned them around to create an opportunity.

When you are able to take a step back and think about the journey you are on and realise it's an experience that can either propel you forwards or backwards depending on your perception, that's an incredibly powerful place to be.

It takes you from the position of victim to victor and allows you to reclaim control of your life and destiny. And when you can do that, your whole world opens up.

CHAPTER THREE

THE MONUMENTAL MUCK-UP OF MODERN MEDICINE

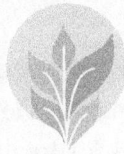

Now that you are familiar with our background story, what we're about to reveal in this chapter may not come as a surprise. Time and time again, we are left baffled and bewildered at the extent to which we are being let down by modern (conventional) medicine.

It's important to understand how the medical system operates because we are then able to understand why the solutions offered by this system don't provide the results we need. We must acknowledge why pills and potions don't truly fix our health conditions and why the gene blame game discourages individuals from taking ownership of their health.

When we are able to look beyond what is truly going on within our medical system and see past the fancy trends and savvy marketing ploys, we can then put our hands back on the steering wheel and take control of our health and wellbeing.

Shockingly, the majority of our clients come to us when they are at their wits end. They are stuck, frustrated and confused after spending years of their lives and thousands of precious dollars going to doctors and specialists who they trust to deliver them reliable answers.

Most of the time, they walk away with nothing other than packets of pills and a feeling of being unheard.

We need to address these issues because too many people are putting their trust in a system that is letting them down. Too many people are being medicated for health issues that for the most part, have an alternative and safer solution. We have a society of chronically sick people who believe they are at the mercy of their genes and are getting sucked into the latest piece of 'scientific' research.

Ultimately, we need to blow the cover off the truth on how we can heal.

In this chapter, we uncover the real reasons behind why we are so sick; why those pills on your kitchen bench aren't your friends, how your DNA does not determine your destiny, why we need to be wary of the latest fads and trends and how we can move forward with a holistic approach to our health.

Great Doctors, Poor System

Let's be clear; we are not blaming doctors when we talk about the muck-up of modern medicine. We think doctors are amazing and dedicated people who more often than not have a deep desire to help people. Why would you enter the tough world of medicine if making a positive different wasn't your driving force?

Over our lifetimes, we've both had our fair share of incredible support from doctors and specialists who we believe are working to the best of their ability within the system they are entrenched. The overwhelming majority of doctors are caring, professional and carry out their role with admirable expertise.

What we have come to understand – through our own experiences and witnessing those of our clients – is that conventional medicine is fantastic for dealing with acute illness and trauma but not so good for chronic illness.

By acute illness and trauma, we mean events such as a sudden heart attack or stroke, or a head injury from a serious car accident. These sudden events are easily diagnosed, there's little confusion around what caused them and trained professionals are able to perform routine surgeries and procedures to save lives. Medical technology is so advanced that patients are often able to make incredible recoveries from what are life-threatening events.

Chronic illness, on the other hand, is a long-term condition with ongoing symptoms that lessen one's quality of life over a period of time. Often there's not one clear trigger – or the causes of symptoms aren't always obvious. Examples include conditions such as lupus, chronic fatigue syndrome, anxiety, depression, migraines, thyroid disorder, type-2 diabetes leaky gut syndrome, heart palpitations and autoimmune disease.

The truth is, many long-term health conditions are still a source of mystery within the conventional medical field because practitioners are limited to working only with the information that science and research can provide.

While technology and science are advancing at a rapid pace, we only know what we know and until we can know every single thing about the thousands of intricacies within the human body, there will still be a guessing game going on to some degree in your doctor's office. Unfortunately, the result of a doctor not knowing an answer can lead to a devastating result; denial or even misdiagnosis.

Have you ever heard of somebody's symptoms being diagnosed as psychosomatic, where the recommendation is to go and see a psychiatrist? Or where the doctor may dismiss their very real symptoms by telling them they are bored or overworked and they need meditation or a new hobby?

Who on earth has the time, energy or desire to dream up a whole raft of imaginary symptoms and then take themselves off to the doctor to go through the lengthy process of having symptoms that don't even exist diagnosed?

Can you imagine the frustration and despair of a patient who is experiencing very real pain or discomfort, then being told, it's all in their heads?

Unbelievably, this diagnosis is still being handed out to this day – because doctors simply don't have all the answers. It's easier to dismiss the patient and blame their symptoms on an over-reactive imagination than to admit they can't give an accurate diagnosis.

Steve has witnessed this first-hand with his mother. Before she was diagnosed with CFS, she was told her symptoms were imaginary. We've seen several other examples of misdiagnosis with our clients over the years. One example is a recent client with CFS who was told he needed to see a psychiatrist. It's time to call out these misdiagnoses and expose them for what they are; complete rubbish.

Remember, we are not criticising the doctors. Misdiagnoses are happening because we are not yet at a point technologically where they can know everything about the human body. Also, the funding to produce the research we need is often lacking, or trends redirect studies in another direction. It's only a matter of time before the correct diagnostic technology will be available – but in the meantime, incorrect diagnoses such as, *"It's all in your head,"* are still very much a reality.

Women in particular are suffering the effects of this misdiagnosis.

Overall, women are becoming sicker and sicker to an extent that can't be ignored, so doctors are eager to hand out a diagnosis – even if it's wrong. It's no wonder we have a society where an increasing number of people are unwell and unhappy. Their health is plummeting and they have no idea what to do about it.

Epstein-Barr Virus

Viral and pathogenic activity in the body is a relatively new area of natural medicine that we have started to delve into which is proving incredibly powerful at preventing and reversing chronic illness and forms a component of our coaching programmes. That is the exploration of the Epstein-Barr virus as the root cause of many (if not most) of the health conditions we see today in modern society.

This virus is known about within conventional medicine, but not a lot of attention has been given to it. The theory behind the Epstein-Barr virus is that it has several different strains and the degree of an individual's illness can be linked back to the severity of the particular strain. The virus can be handed down through the bloodline from our parents and can be transmitted very easily from person to person.

The over-prescription of medications such as antibiotics causes the virus to mutate, become antibiotic resistant and harder to remove from the body. It thrives on things like toxic heavy metals in the body and certain everyday foods – many of which we are told are good for us. The virus replicates and defecates in the body, creating a by-product that creates aggressive and nasty symptoms such as brain fog, pain, insomnia, night sweats, hot flushes, tingling hands, numbness, dizziness, vertigo, chest pain, asthma, fatigue, fibromyalgia, moodiness, confusion, anxiety and PTSD.

If you've ever had glandular fever (known as mononucleosis in the USA), we know you have a severe strain of the Epstein-Barr virus in your body. The virus can lie dormant in the organs (particularly the liver) then unleash itself when the immune system is low, such as during times of stress and hormonal change – which is why women are hit particularly hard with symptoms.

It feeds off emotions such as fear and worry as these lower the immune system and allow the virus to replicate itself and attack the body. There are multiple triggers for the virus to begin an attack.

Most varieties of the virus can be removed within roughly one year if you are patient, focus on a low-stress lifestyle and consume healing foods that will kill the virus and prevent the replication of new virus cells. This subject is too broad to cover here but is something we go into in more detail in our coaching programmes.

The Body Does Not Attack Itself

Conventional medicine will have us believe that autoimmune dysfunction is the result of the body attacking itself. Alternative and holistic medicine takes a very different view.

We are born into these incredible machines with the capacity to heal and thrive on a daily basis. Our bodies fight every single day to keep us well and ensure all functions work as they should. Anyone who has ever been sick and then recovered will know that their body did so innately, without being asked.

Why would one's body then suddenly start to attack itself? It makes no sense.

This theory is very disempowering because people begin to think they don't have any control over their health and that they are at the mercy of a faulty body. It removes the belief and motivation required to heal.

This approach is quite frankly, a total and utter disaster.

Our methods prove that, contrary to attacking itself, the body is desperate to be well and will do anything to be well. We have seen dozens and dozens of our clients reverse their autoimmune conditions once we explain this misguided theory, address the true cause of illness in the body and provide them with the tools and support to recover.

Medication is Not a Fix

Modern day medical training is based around diagnosing symptoms, then offering medication as a 'fix.' Medication only masks symptoms though, it never addresses the root cause. Then, of course, there is the risk of developing side effects from the medication, thereby requiring further medication to address the side effects. It's essentially a merry-go-round with no exit!

This approach also trains us to believe that we need pills and potions to fix our sick bodies, rather than empowering the individual to take control of their own state of health. This is a source of endless frustration for us because we can see the trap society has fallen into. We have a population of sick people being kept alive by medication because they are offered no alternative solution.

Hippocrates, known as the Father of Medicine, lived in the years between 460 BC and 375 BC and taught that all forms of illness have a natural cause. He is well known for his famous quote, *"Let food be thy medicine, and medicine be thy food."*

Yet in the years that followed, conventional medicine has deviated so far from that approach that food is considered completely irrelevant to our state of health.

In fact, nutritional training in medical school is incredibly limited and mainly based on bio-medical factors, such as how protein is metabolised in the body. Medical students are not taught how nutrition plays a role in the prevention and treatment of disease.

We know on a personal level – but also from working with our clients – that food is so fundamental to the overall state of one's health that we find it unbelievable that its importance is not acknowledged in the medical field.

It also blows our mind that someone who lived thousands of years ago, before any kind of technology existed, had it so right, yet today, we've got it all so wrong.

We understand why our medical system is not set up to deal with chronic illness. As already mentioned, it's partly because science and research have not yet delivered all the answers. Another reason is the massive influence on our medical system by the pharmaceutical industry.

Have you ever thought about how much money pharmaceutical companies turn over? And have you ever considered what would happen to all those profits if we had a wonderfully healthy population?

Makes you think, doesn't it?

The truth is, the pharmaceutical industry holds an immense amount of power over the way our medical system operates.

This puts sick patients at a disadvantage because they are being brainwashed into believing that medication is the only answer to all their problems. How disempowering is that – to know that you are reliant on a pill or drug to help you feel better?

Sometimes, we have a real urge to march into the hospital waiting rooms and shout, *"No! Here is a better way! You can be well again! You don't need all the pills! Come with us and we'll show you how!"*

We know that 95% of the time, we could give those patients a six-week programme that would completely turn their health around based on some very simple yet fundamental principles.

We are aware that many people just want to take the easy road and take a pill. They don't want to do the work of adjusting their lifestyle or paying closer attention to what they're putting in their mouths. These people will always exist and that's their choice.

But we believe that there are millions of people out there who wouldn't rely on medication if they knew there was another way, who would want to get to the bottom of the real issue and sort it out for good.

Our mission as holistic health coaches is to bring that message to the fore and show people that there is another way to heal – and it's well within their grasp.

Genetics and Epigenetics

How many times have you heard somebody say they are concerned about getting cancer or dying of heart disease or developing Multiple Sclerosis because that's what their father or aunt or grandmother succumbed to? Or this little nugget, *"Being overweight is in my genes so I'm stuck with it."*

Just because you may be born with certain genes that make you susceptible to a certain disease, doesn't mean you'll end up with it. It's actually your lifestyle choices that will determine whether you develop that disease up to 95% of the time.

Your destiny is not determined by your family history; contrary to what conventional medicine might be telling us.

A relatively new and fascinating field of medicine called epigenetics studies the control of gene activity. In simple terms, it's the study of how your lifestyle choices and behaviours can influence the way in which your genes work and how they are expressed.

For example, twins separated at birth have the same DNA sequence but will end up with different diseases dependent on their choice of lifestyle. If the father of these twins died of a heart attack and each twin inherited 50% of their DNA from either parent, they would have inherited some susceptibility that they would follow the same fate as their father. Even with exactly the same DNA, one twin could die of a heart attack while the other lived a full and healthy life – all depending on their lifestyle choices.

Lifestyle choices such as following a healthy diet, getting regular exercise, not smoking, keeping stress levels down and drinking little or no alcohol can effectively 'turn off' the 'dodgy' genes you inherited from your parents.

The field of epigenetics is pretty exciting because it empowers us as individuals to know that we are in control of our health. We are not destined for a certain chronic disease just because a family member or two developed it.

By making sensible choices around our lifestyle and behaviours, we can influence our gene expression. So, the next time someone tells you about their health destiny based on genetics, you can reassure them that they are not doomed and can in fact take control of their health.

Fads and Trends

Another area in which society is being let down in the area of health is through fads and trends. These are not limited to the conventional medical field either; they are popping up in alternative medicine as well. Not a week goes by that we don't read or hear about a new health craze that has taken the world by storm. Health drinks, collagen, coffee enemas, oxygen shots, the Keto diet, infrared saunas, the low FODMAP diet, hay bathing (yes, you read that right)... the list goes on and on.

Most fads and trends become popular because of the power and money behind them, not because they actually work. Clever catchphrases and the thought processes they evoke in customers, along with the vested interests driving the trend have a lot more sway over someone's consciousness than any real benefits or results.

Fads and trends also easily attract followers if those who are fronting them paint a beautiful picture of how life could be if you just buy the latest product. We don't think about the fact that the influencer might be 25 years old with no real responsibilities or stressors and hasn't had a health crisis yet.

Images of glowing health, youth and beauty are alluring and it's easy for people to get swept up in the fantasy of it all. We start to believe that this particular product might be just the answer we are looking for – whereas in reality, it most likely isn't.

The danger for those who are struggling with very real symptoms and conditions is they end up questioning their own capabilities and commitment when they don't achieve the promised outcome. Widespread and catchy marketing can end up over-riding common sense and we've seen examples of that several times in the past, particularly when a famous celebrity is involved.

Do you remember the 'appetite suppressant lollipops' endorsed by Kim Kardashian?

Common sense tells us that a hardboiled ball of sugar will not suppress the appetite, yet we get swept away by the promise of a quick fix delivered by a popular influencer. As my wise old Dad always says, *"If it sounds too good to be true, it probably is."*

At the end of the day, trends and fads will not deliver the answers we are looking for and should be treated with extreme caution.

If you are someone who has a deep trust in our medical system because your doctor is highly educated and you believe he or she has the wellspring of information pertaining to your health, you might be feeling a little sceptical by what we have to say. We understand that and we respect your right to make up your own mind.

If you have a health condition that you are struggling to manage, or you are living with symptoms that lessen your quality of life, we ask you to think about how many years and dollars you have spent on trying to fix the problem and whether you are really making progress towards a healthy body and mind.

If the respective answers are 'too many' and 'no', we encourage you to be open-minded to what we are going to share with you in the following chapters.

You may have been led to believe that you are doomed because all your family members are dying prematurely of chronic disease. If you choose to continue with this belief, you will be doing yourself a huge disservice because ultimately, you will fail to take control of your own wellbeing. Think about what it could mean for you if you tossed this belief aside and took ownership of your right to vibrant health.

Being drawn towards the next big shiny solution to your problems is not the answer. Save yourself the money and heartache and stay away from promises delivered by big budgets, clever marketing tactics and glowing faces. A quick fix or the latest trend will not deliver what you are ultimately looking for.

Now that you have a clearer understanding of why you are unwell and why you have been unable to solve your health issues to date, it's time to sink your teeth into mapping out your path forward.

We are going to guide you through a sensible, safe and exceptionally successful approach to how you can recover, heal and start to thrive. All we ask is that you open your mind and trust us, because not only have thousands of our clients walked this path before you, but we also want nothing more than to see you set yourself free.

CHAPTER FOUR

OUR REVOLUTIONARY HEALTH BLUEPRINT

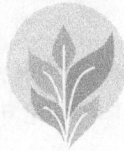

There are two types of people in this world; those with a fixed mindset and those with a growth mindset. We know you have a growth mindset, because those with fixed mindsets don't read books like this.

With a growth mindset, you're already 80% of the way to becoming the best version of you, because you're prepared to learn, discover and grow. The whole purpose of this book is to provide you with the other 20%; our blueprint of how you can reclaim your health, vitality and happiness.

We have a very unique approach to healing which combines equal portions of science, common sense and life experience. This means our methods can't be googled, bought or copied, and it's our own special recipe that can't be offered by anyone else. We are not afraid to say that we have a system that works and we are very proud of it.

For you to trust us, you need to see who we are as people and the philosophies that make up our coaching practice. It's critically important for us to share our message because as you've already discovered, our medical system is creating a society of individuals whose bodies are sick, tired, worn down and pulling on the handbrake in the form of chronic illness and disease.

There is a way to escape from being ruled by this system, *but you have to know how to do it.*

Our revolutionary blueprint will show you how to move away from a slow death and towards a fulfilling and healthy life.

It's also imperative for us to be able to provide guidance to our children and grandchildren because it's well known that for the first time in history, many parents are expected to outlive their children due to obesity and poor health.

> *"Atherosclerosis, hardening of the arteries, begins in childhood. By age 10, nearly all kids have fatty streaks, the first stage of the disease."*
>
> (Dr Michael Greger, Author of How Not to Die)

There is a very real danger in not understanding how to remove yourself (and your family) from the trap of conventional medicine. You risk living your life with a body and mind that isn't given the opportunity to function as it's designed to.

Who wants to stay stuck in first gear because it's too difficult to go any further?

Our bodies are incredibly intelligent machines that strive to be well. What an absolute tragedy and disservice we are doing to ourselves.

Below, we are going to discuss what areas of natural medicine we specialise in, the coaching philosophies we live by personally and encourage you to follow and how to get started on creating positive, straightforward changes that have the power to change your life.

Natural Medicine

Our interest in natural medicine came about out of necessity because conventional medicine failed me, as outlined earlier. A medicine designed to 'help' me actually did the reverse and sent me to a place of utter despair.

Our experience is not unique, but is happening on a global scale – particularly with potent medications such as steroids. Not only are these medications not addressing the root cause of the health issue, they are causing dreadful side effects. In order for me to recover, we had no choice but to investigate alternatives, which led us down the path of holistic health.

Together, we bring a unique set of skills and life experience to deliver an exceptionally successful coaching programme to our clients, focusing on the five pillars of health: *Nutrition, exercise, gut health, sleep and addressing the root cause of stress.*

We focus on everything from using food, exercise and pre-bed routines to personal coaching techniques to reduce stress and balance hormones, assess the way we perceive certain situations and maintain or improve healthy adrenal gland function.

Walking the Talk

We are very careful to make sure we 'walk the talk' and would never ask a client to do anything we haven't tried ourselves. Often, we will come across a new theory or something that makes sense and we will test it out first before offering it as an option to our clients.

We are very open and honest about our background story and will happily share the gory details because it's important for our clients to know that we are coaching from a place of first-hand experience. We are also very honest about how we live our lives. It's in nobody's interest to think we've got it all sorted and that we live perfect lives with perfect health at all times. That is so far from the truth!

We talk a lot about the 80/20 rule; 80% of the time make good choices and 20% of the time, let your hair down and do what you like. Who wants to follow a rigid plan at all times and have no life? Not us!

That's why you'll see Steve cracking open a craft beer or two and me popping open a bag of jellybeans occasionally. We have cheat meals and we go to bed late sometimes and we're very open about it. If we weren't, we'd be lying by omission of the facts.

We live a very normal life, but we do put a lot of focus on our health and wellbeing. We are more interested in making sure we have a stash of frozen mango in the freezer and a block of dark chocolate in the pantry than we are about planning our next overseas holiday.

That's the truth!

We have found that when our bodies are humming nicely physically and mentally, those desires for all the external flash and fancy things in life start to subside, because there's a general feeling of internal contentment.

We are honest with people because we want them to be honest with us and comfortable to tell us about the choices they make and when they slip up. So you slipped up? Who cares? Just get back on track the next day and move on. Easy.

We don't make things harder than they need to be.

Health is Wealth

Isn't it interesting how as a society we are so focused on building our assets and wealth, yet we forget about the most valuable asset we will ever own; our health. We spend our hard-earned cash on houses and cars and all the trappings of a 'comfortable' life, yet many of us are uncomfortably residing in a body that is struggling.

Occasionally, we will have a client who doesn't want to invest the money in our services to get them back on track. When we start breaking down the cost of what they're spending on things like alcohol, takeaways and fancy coffees each week, it becomes clear that the cost of the programme is not the real issue. The real issue is that they don't view their health as a top priority or investment.

Think about all the money you've spent over the years on visits to doctors, specialists, gimmicks or interesting-looking creams or potions that you think will help you feel better. Has the investment been worth it? Or are you still stuck in the same pattern of going round and round in circles with ongoing symptoms and rounds of medications that make you feel lousy?

Could that money have been better spent by focusing on the things that will actually work, such as whole, nutrient-dense foods or a mentor with proven results who can help you get your spark back?

Another thing to consider is that those little niggles, aches and pains or perhaps something more serious will not magically disappear as the years tick by. You can be sure that symptoms will generally worsen with the natural ageing process.

That extra 15kg you're holding onto right now? That thyroid issue that is bugging you? Your high blood-pressure reading? None of these things are going to miraculously disappear into thin air over the course of the next weeks, months and years.

Chances are, in another 10 years, they will be worse than they are right now and in another 20 years, they could be debilitating. Unless, of course, you take control and start treating your health as your most important and valuable asset.

Listen to Your Gut

We're big on this one! Our intuition, or gut instinct, is super important and often overlooked. How many times has something happened in your life, or you've done something, then looked back and said, *"I knew I shouldn't have done that, but I did it anyway."*

We've all been there.

That's our gut instinct telling us that what we're about to do is not in our best interests, but because we let our brains or hearts take over, we end up doing something we regret. Our gut instinct is actually our sixth sense and it must never be ignored. It can appear in several different ways and is unique to each individual, such as a churning or sick feeling in the tummy, alarm bells in your head or a red flag popping up in your mind's eye.

The reason we talk about gut instinct a lot with our clients is because we've experienced first-hand how important it is. When I was very sick, Steve would often check in to see what his gut was saying. His gut told him that I would be okay and that we would get through it.

This is one of the reasons he was able to shoulder such a huge responsibility of running our business, caring for me, the kids and looking after the household. His gut was telling him everything was going to work out okay in the end, so he was then able to focus on what needed to be done and get on with doing it, rather than endlessly worrying and fretting.

The true test of whether you are in sync with your gut instinct is to check in with your anxiety levels. The gut-brain connection is incredibly strong and a disconnect with your gut instinct can result in worry and anxiety. If you are constantly fretting or on high alert, it's a sign that there are problems with your gut and therefore your gut instinct will be in a state of misalignment.

A settled mind will enable you to sit quietly and check in with your gut instinct when necessary. It is there to protect you and will never let you down.

Lead by Example

Making changes in life can be challenging because the people around you won't necessarily understand what you're doing and sometimes they won't like it. When you start seeing great results from your efforts and start feeling better, it's tempting to shout from the rooftops about what you're doing and convince everyone else they should be doing the same. Very rarely is this approach effective.

Other people don't like to be told what to do, and they certainly don't like their current failings being highlighted by someone who suddenly has all the answers!

Frequently our clients will tell us that they have been sharing with their friends and family how wonderful they are feeling and that they are encouraging the people around them to copy what they're doing.

In this situation, we remind them that the best possible thing they can do is lead by example. Even if they think they are offering encouragement, it can come across as being preachy or putting the pressure on and the response can be less than favourable.

Leading by example is about quietly going about your business and doing what you need to do to focus on yourself and your health, then watching the flow-on effects to the people around you. When they notice a difference in the way you look or carry yourself, or how you seem calmer or happier, they will naturally become curious and want to know what you're doing. When they show interest, they are more likely to be open-minded and receptive to what you tell them.

We've seen examples of this within our own close circle of family and friends. Someone will be dealing with a certain health condition and will decide to take control and make positive changes.

After a period of time, others will notice the positive change in that person and think to themselves that maybe they should look at doing something similar. This creates a flow-on effect to other members in the group and is far more effective than trying to convince someone to do something they're not ready for.

If Something Isn't Working, Change It

There's a well-known saying that the definition of insanity is doing the same thing over and over again and expecting different results. This is a common theme we see with our clients (no we're not calling them insane!), when they are trying to change habits, lose weight or get on top of their health problems. They have good intentions to stick with their goals and follow through, but when things get tough, they naturally default back to their old patterns, then wonder why nothing ever works.

We see people who have spent years of their lives and thousands of dollars pursuing potential remedies that don't offer them the results they are looking for. Because we are conditioned to believe that doctors and conventional medicine have all the answers, we blindly follow that path with high hopes. Well, now we know that conventional medicine doesn't have all the answers and can be a bit like the blind leading the blind in some cases.

If this sounds like you and you have no idea what to do next, we are here to tell you that if what you are doing isn't working, you must do something completely different. And that's where we come in!

We've done the hard work and paved the way for you. What has taken us years and years to figure out is now condensed into an easy-to-follow programme to get your health in tip-top shape. There's no need to keep going around in circles repeating the things you've always done and wondering why there's not a different outcome.

You may need to challenge your beliefs or behaviours to get you the results you desire.

A lifetime of habitual patterns can be tricky to undo, especially if you subconsciously aren't willing to change them.

For example, you eat eggs every morning for breakfast and you can't live without them? Well, they may be making you sick, so are you going to keep defending your wish to eat eggs? Can you accept that eggs have led to a state of disease that you're no longer willing to live with? Or will you continue to eat the eggs and expect to become well? Don't expect to keep doing the same old thing and generate different results.

This ties in nicely with our philosophy on making sustainable lifestyle changes. We don't endorse diets or quick fixes that promise the world because we've been in the industry long enough to know these pathways lead to disappointment and frustration.

A sustainable lifestyle change is about simple changes to one's lifestyle that are easy to sustain over the long term. It is a sensible and effective approach to addressing health issues because it heals the body from the inside out over time – and you might be surprised at how quickly your health can be turned around for the better when you start following a common-sense approach.

We don't believe in deprivation or telling you not to eat a certain food ever again. We want you to have a life and we want you to enjoy it! That means being able to go out for dinner on a special occasion, have dessert and a couple of glasses of wine and enjoy every moment.

We teach you how to enjoy these times, erase the guilt, then get back to healthy habits the next day. It's super easy and a big part of the reason our clients are able to maintain a great state of health long after they have finished working with us.

Finding Purpose

We've shared with you how we were able to take our respective challenging experiences, identify the reason for going through them and flip them around to create a purpose. That purpose is to spread our health philosophy far and wide and help our clients transform their lives for the better. We now teach others how to rearrange their mindset to enable them to find their reasons and purpose.

When our clients are feeling down on their luck and that life is an uphill slog, we have our own quote we like to share with them:

"When you turn 'why me' into 'this is why', everything changes and the whole world opens up."

(Heidi and Steve Jennings)

In other words, when you adjust your thinking patterns from being a victim to finding a reason for your suffering, you go from a negative mindset to a positive one and when this happens, the world is your oyster.

We understand the natural hesitation people have in following our approach when they may have been burned many times in the past with methods that haven't worked. Personally, we spent years and thousands of dollars on doctors, naturopaths and various medications and supplements to address my eczema over the years, so we get it.

If you are in this position, we encourage you to be open minded and take a common-sense approach. Masking symptoms through medication will never heal your body and allow you to experience vibrant health and vitality. It's critical to start addressing the root cause of the problems and the only way to do that is to allow the body to heal via natural medicine that actually works.

We have done this with thousands of clients and 95% of the time, their lives are completely transformed. By all means, do your due diligence and listen to what your gut instinct is telling you. Does it feel right to keep doing what you've been doing? Or does it make more sense to change it?

Perhaps you are doubting your commitment or ability to focus on something new because you've never been able to stick to anything in the past. When you take a common-sense approach, stickability becomes less of an issue because the changes required are straightforward and easy to implement. You won't feel like you're missing out on anything and within a very short space of time, you'll start to feel so much better that reverting back to old habits will become very unappealing.

Of course, there is an element of discipline required but we assure you will be pleasantly surprised at how easy our methods are to follow.

You may be thinking, *"Well, if the natural health approach is so simple and sensible, why isn't everyone doing it already?"*

Great question. Human beings have a habit of making things a lot more complicated than they need to be.

We could all just eat nutritious food, do some exercise, look after our gut, get lots of sleep and learn how to manage our stress better, couldn't we? But no, we stuff 'food' loaded with preservatives, additives, artificial flavourings and colourings into our mouths and wash it down with soft drink or alcohol. We slog ourselves senseless at the gym to work off all the crap food and drink. We annihilate any beneficial gut bacteria to ensure we have a festering mess of a gut and therefore, mental health problems. We go to bed at midnight and put ourselves on the back foot for the next day.

And we do all of these things to exacerbate the general stress that goes along with living on this earth, just to make life ten times more stressful than it has to be.

As a society we have moved so far away from common sense it's not even funny. What we're doing to ourselves is actually very sad because all we really need to do is take a step back, simplify our habits and choices and watch our lives transform before our eyes.

Remember, that's not in the interests of the powerful pharmaceutical companies, is it?

The reality is, we've been sucked into a medical system that is slowly killing us.

So, let's change that. It's time to delve into the nitty gritty of the five pillars of health that will completely transform your health and your life.

CHAPTER FIVE

NAIL YOUR NUTRITION

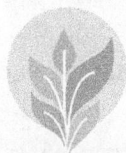

The first of our five pillars is nutrition and it's a very important one. The right nutrition has the power to completely change the way you look, feel and show up in the world. The way most people are showing up in the world (sluggish, sad and sick) indicates that our nutritional habits are way off the mark and need some serious attention.

The fact is, the way our society is eating is leading us towards a slow death. You might think this sounds dramatic, but out of our 10 top causes of death, seven are directly related to nutrition.* The rich and powerful food industry is often a minefield of corruption, contradiction and confusion and we are stuck smack bang in the middle of it.

There are things we definitely should not be eating and things we definitely should be eating more of, but no-one is very clear on what those things are. Instead, we are utterly confused because things have become over-complicated and we are constantly bombarded by 'scientific studies' that end up contradicting themselves time and time again.

We desperately need the right knowledge to enable us to step away from the corruption and confusion.

Without the knowledge we are going to share with you, you are at risk of continuing along this dangerous path, eating all those foods you have been told are good for you but are actually very damaging. You are at risk of being stuck in a vicious cycle of never-ending confusion around what is healthy and what isn't.

This can easily lead to the trap of yo-yo diets, calorie counting, macronutrient obsession and buying into the next gimmick or fad, simply because you are clutching at straws and really have no idea who or what to believe. Worst of all, without the right knowledge, you are at a loss in knowing how to heal your body and live the healthy, happy life you deserve.

The majority of our clients are either very confused about what they should be eating or are convinced they are eating fairly well. When we point out what role some of those 'healthy' foods are playing in their poor state of health, they are often shocked.

"The problem with the Standard American Diet (SAD), a primary cause of the current obesity epidemic, is the fact that the majority of foods consumed are high in calories, and low in macronutrients."

(Dr Joel Fuhrman)

In this chapter, we are going to delve into how our habits surrounding food are leading to a sick population, which foods are making you sick, how to empower yourself with the right food and how to get off the diet merry-go-round for good.

Back in the good old days, humans ate what they could hunt and gather from their surrounding environment. Their diet consisted of things like various meats, fruits and vegetables, nuts and seeds and honey. Today, our version of hunting and gathering is walking into a huge supermarket, wandering the aisles and plonking all sorts of cardboard boxes and packets full of factory-made 'food' into our trolleys. And somewhere in between, we went from a population of lean, fit and healthy individuals to one of obese, sick and unhappy ones. What on earth went wrong?

Let's jump into that rabbit hole and find out about some of the things that are making us sick.

Food Addiction

Processed and refined foods loaded with salt, fat, sugar and gluten are very addictive because they trigger neurons in the brain. They are devoid of any real nutrients and are designed to make us hungry, so we end up eating more than we should, fuelling the addiction, cravings and a loss of self-control.

Almost everyone has a form of food addiction these days. Not you? Think about the biscuit you need with your cup of tea, the coffee first thing in the morning, the wine before dinner, the salt and vinegar chips at 3pm or the energy drinks to get you through until your next cup of coffee. These are all habits that lead to addictive tendencies.

Sugar

Sugar triggers dopamine in the brain, is highly addictive and its effect on the brain has been likened to cocaine. It's regularly added to highly processed foods, leading to the average adult consuming over 20 teaspoons per day. It weakens our immune systems and creates the ideal environment for cancer growth, diabetes, obesity, mental illness, autoimmune conditions and heart disease.

Gluten

Gluten is highly problematic in the human body because it contains toxic and damaging proteins. It is in almost every type of food, including those you least expect, such as gravy and chewing gum. Long-term consumption of gluten damages the intestinal lining, weakens the bowel and hinders the absorption of food.

Sooner or later, if you're eating gluten on a regular basis, your body may start to rebel, resulting in inflammatory bowel and colon diseases such as colitis, diverticulitis and Irritable Bowel Syndrome (IBS). Other symptoms of gluten sensitivity include stomach aches, constipation, diarrhoea, bloating, gall bladder disease, liver disease, chronic fatigue, osteoporosis, headaches, irritability, among many, many others.

Dairy

Dairy products contain high levels of fat and are extremely difficult for your intestines and liver to process. They are also highly inflammatory and provide an ideal food source for viral and pathogenic activity in the body. Casein in milk has been proven to be carcinogenic (cancer-causing) and lactose creates a food source for viruses and pathogens, leading to inflammation, allergies and mucus.

Dairy is problematic for everyone, even though you may not necessarily display symptoms. If you are someone who experiences joint pain or general aches and pains in the body, or you cough up a lot of mucus and have to clear your throat before you speak, you'll be amazed at what removing dairy from your diet will do. And don't worry about not getting enough calcium if you don't eat dairy.

It's a myth that we need dairy products to build strong bones. Why, when New Zealanders are one of the largest consumers of dairy in the world, do we have one of the highest rates of osteoporosis? A bit odd, don't you think?

Meat

Even lean cuts of meat are high in saturated fat and place a burden on the liver. Meat also strips the gut of hydrochloric acid, an essential stomach acid that helps to break down, digest and absorb nutrients. Long term studies on the intake of animal protein show detrimental effects to health and stress on the kidneys and bones. If you like to eat meat, we recommend no more than a palm-sized piece of animal protein per day, and even less if possible.

Low Carbohydrate Diets

Low-carb diets have been a huge trend in recent years but they simply don't work. Carbs are normally the main source of sugar in the bloodstream and therefore our primary source of fuel. Things start to go haywire when we limit our intake.

If carbohydrate intake is too low, your adrenaline hormone tends to rise to meet the demands of your busy schedule. When this happens, you stop burning fat, become edgy, irritable, may not sleep well and eventually you'll crave salty or sweet carb-dense foods.

This craving is your body's way of saying, *"Give me more fuel to meet the demands of our hectic schedule!"*

This is where an emotional relationship with food kicks in. You get stressed or busy, your adrenaline rises to keep you alert, you crave carbs to fuel the body, then you overeat the wrong type of foods. This hormonal merry-go-round leads to stubborn bodyfat and ultimately, a rut that can be hard to break free from.

Yes, you can burn fat when you have less carbohydrates in the body, but fat is burned as energy in times of low stress – like walking, yoga or deep sleep. The combination of high stress and low carbs is best avoided.

Low-carb intake also leads to a drop in blood sugar levels, meaning that the adrenal glands have to step in to produce extra cortisol to pull glucose out of your muscles and liver. This creates lower energy levels, sugar cravings and fat storage.

Do yourself a favour and get away from the mindset that 'low carb is good.' It's not and your health will suffer.

Alcohol

Alcohol is a carcinogen that causes a wide range of health conditions and chronic disease. It's a neurotoxin that poisons your organs, disrupts your hormones and is strongly linked to liver disease, breast cancer and a reduction in lifespan. It's full of empty calories and the more you drink, the fatter you get. It's best avoided for optimal health or consumed only rarely in small quantities.

Have you heard that red wine is heart healthy because it contains resveratrol? That's the alcohol industry manipulating you into buying their product. Any benefits from resveratrol in wine is offset by the alcohol content, so if you want to be heart healthy, go directly to the source and eat the grapes instead.

Our society has a real problem with alcohol. Have you seen those funny memes circulating on the internet about the mum who needs a bottle of wine to take the edge off each night? They're not so funny when you uncover how many of those mums (and dads) are actually full-blown alcoholics.

Coffee

Coffee is the most popular drink in the world – and the most addictive. Coffee is very high in caffeine, extremely dehydrating to the body and strips away vital stores of vitamin B, iron and zinc.

Caffeine stimulates the adrenal glands to activate the breakdown and release of liver glycogen, releasing it as blood sugar and giving you an instant shot of energy. The pancreas then excretes higher levels of insulin in an effort to bring blood sugar levels back to normal. Your body then goes into survival mode and leads to your adrenal glands producing more cortisol – the stress and alert hormone.

Every hit of caffeine activates the same response in the body, leading to adrenal glands that get exhausted and worn out over

FROM LIVING HELL TO LIVING WELL

time. It's also a liver loader, raises blood pressure and can lead to obesity because it stimulates cortisol, leading to deadly fat storage around the organs in the abdomen.

For optimal health, coffee should be removed from the diet. We understand though how addictive and enjoyable our coffee rituals can be. For anyone who wants to keep drinking coffee, stick with one cup per day, preferably before 9am.

Fruit Fear

Worryingly, the fear of fruit has become very real. From the beginning of time, we have known that fruit is a necessary component of human health. It is fundamental for building a strong and healthy body and for healing chronic disease.

In the past couple of decades, however, there has been a lot of very misleading – and corrupt – propaganda dispelling the virtues of fruit, to the point that people are fearful of it. Why? Well, there's no money in fruit, is there?

People also get confused about the impacts fruit has on the body. Someone who has been eating the SAD for a long period of time who then starts eating fruit might say, *"Oh, but bananas make me bloated,"* or *"Oh, but apples don't agree with me."*

This is actually not correct. What happens when you eat fruit is that it *strengthens your immune system*. Your immune system then goes to war on all the gunk in the body, in an effort to get rid of it. This can cause unpleasant side effects (temporarily), but it's because your body is fighting disease. Once you get through the initial discomfort, you will find that fruit does actually agree with you.

It is crucial for your health and will supercharge the healing process.

Other Trouble-Makers

There are other foods that trigger and instigate serious health issues which we refer to as 'trouble-makers.' These foods wreak havoc on our health but are often not widely known as such. We have already talked about the view in holistic medicine that most chronic illness is caused by viral and pathogenic activity in the body and that this activity thrives on certain foods.

Health professionals are unlikely to warn you about the dangers of these foods (apart from alcohol), because, as already discussed, conventional medical training does not focus on nutrition as a solution for chronic illness and does not recognise the true impact of the Epstein-Barr virus on our health.

Here are the trouble-makers to be aware of:

- All dairy products (milk, cheese, yoghurt, kefir)
- Gluten
- Soft drinks
- Eggs
- Tuna
- Pork
- Industrial food oils (vegetable/palm/canola/corn/safflower)
- Vinegar
- Fermented foods
- Alcohol
- Aspartame and other artificial sweeteners
- MSG (mono-sodium glutamate)
- Preservatives and additives

Look at that list and think about how often you consume these foods. It's likely you are eating many of them several times a week, if not daily. A lot of our clients are loath to give up eggs, but when we explain to them that eggs are a fuel source for problematic viral activity in the body, they have a crack (excuse the pun!) at giving them up and very quickly realise that their symptoms are starting to disappear – eggs-tremely quickly.

Vinegar and too many fermented foods will pickle your liver, so don't buy into the fermented food craze or be sucked into guzzling gallons of kombucha and adding fermented foods such as kimchi to every meal. A lot of this is about marketing hype and making money, not about giving you good health.

Artificial sugars such as aspartame will strip your gut of beneficial bacteria and can create neurological problems. Dairy products are inflammatory and a proven carcinogen. Tuna is loaded with mercury, a toxic heavy metal which can lodge itself in the organs and also provides a delightful food source for viral activity. MSG is a flavour enhancer often found in foods such as potato chips and is a carcinogen. Oils are loaded with saturated fat and are not heart-healthy, even though they are marketed as such. Soft drinks are packed with so much sugar they should be illegal. Preservatives and additives are man-made chemicals that can damage our health.

None of the foods and drinks in this list are going to give you vibrant health and when you consider that most people eat these foods *all the time,* it's not hard to see why health problems are so prevalent in our society.

Friendly Foods

Now we are aware of the types of foods we should be avoiding, let's take a look at the foods that will make us want to scale buildings in a single bound! These are the foods we absolutely must start paying attention to and bringing into our lives if we want to live inside a happy and healthy body.

Below is a list of the foods to introduce for optimal health and wellness:

- All fruit (fresh, frozen, dried)
- All vegetables, especially leafy greens
- Whole grains (focus on simple and complex, not refined carbohydrates)
- Legumes
- Nuts
- Seeds

These are whole, nutrient-dense foods that will provide the body with the goodness it needs. When you start eating the way nature intended, your body will naturally start to recalibrate and the healing process can initiate. Cravings will subside because vitamin and mineral requirements are being met and you will find the swings and roundabouts of yo-yo dieting will naturally fade into oblivion.

Giving your body what it needs and nothing more is a powerful place to be. No more confusion about what and when to eat and no more worrying about calories and portion sizes equates to absolute freedom and will completely change your life.

Let's not forget the importance of drinking plenty of water. It's not always the easiest or most pleasant thing to do, but it is super important! Water delivers oxygen, nutrients and waste to and from your organs and cells. It helps regulate body temperature and protects your joints, tissues and organs from damage and shock. Ideally, adults should consume 2 – 2.5 litres of water every day to stay hydrated and to allow for optimal physical and mental performance. A good way to know if you are well hydrated is to check your urine; it should run clear.

A Healing Crisis

When you start making positive changes to your diet, the body can start to heal and you will notice changes in your physical and mental state. Don't be concerned if you go through some initial detoxification symptoms. These can vary from person to person but will typically include things like aches and pains, general lethargy or cold and flu symptoms.

Often, your most prominent health issue can flare up during detoxification. For example, somebody with regular migraines might find their migraines get temporarily worse. Eating the 'friendly foods' mentioned above strengthen your immune system, which then has the capacity to attack and dispel all the toxins and gunk out of the dark depths of the body. This can result in temporary discomfort as these toxins are activated and eliminated.

This is sometimes referred to as a 'healing crisis' and is a sign that your body is doing what it is designed to do – protect you and keep you well. Also, it's important to understand that healing is not always a linear process, even though we expect it to be. In some cases, it can be more of a 'three steps forward, two steps back' process, but be assured that your body knows exactly what it is doing and will heal in its own time, given the right support.

Supplementation

We are big believers in obtaining all the vitamins and minerals we need from our food, however, with our busy modern-day lifestyles and deteriorating soil quality, this isn't always achievable. There are four main supplements we recommend to our clients to support the healing process and overall good health. These are listed below, with a brief summary of benefits for each:

- Vitamin B12 – antiviral, supports liver function, central nervous system and brain.
- Liquid Zinc Sulfate – antiviral, supports liver function, skin and wound healing, sexual function, insulin and growth hormones.
- Spirulina powder – prevents viral/bacterial growth inside the liver, prevents iron deficiency, supports toxic heavy metal detox and liver detox.
- Barley grass powder – beneficial for stomach issues, gout and arthritis, feeds the liver and is a potent toxic heavy metal detoxifier.

Fasting

While there is plenty of research showing the benefits of fasting, a word of caution here. Fasting is fine for people who are generally healthy and feeling good most of the time and can be a great tool for weight loss.

If you are someone who has a very busy lifestyle, feels stressed or overwhelmed – or has a lot of underlying health issues – fasting can cause more harm than good. This is because a drop in carbohydrate intake stimulates the release of adrenaline to help the body cope with the lack of available glucose (the body's source of fuel). Too much adrenaline can push the body into further distress.

Know What's in Your Food

We must highlight the importance of educating yourself on what is in your food. It's inevitable in our busy world that we will still rely on processed and packaged food to some extent (kudos to you if you don't!) and as such, it's a very good idea to know what all those mysterious letters and numbers on the packaging of food products actually mean.

Many food companies label their foods as 'healthy' when in fact they are packed full of fat, sugar, gluten, animal meats and fats, additives, preservatives and artificial colourings and flavourings. None of these things are beneficial for human health.

Many years ago when I became aware of my food sensitivities, I spent a lot of time educating myself on how to read nutrition labels. I had to be aware of all the sneaky ingredients contained in foods to be able to eliminate those that were causing my eczema.

I remember the day I asked Steve to look after the kids while I went to the supermarket and spent about two hours walking up and down the aisles, taking packets off shelves, reading and interpreting them.

That was such an important investment of my time because it opened my eyes to what was really in the common, everyday foods I had been purchasing regularly. Each time I went to the supermarket after that, I was able to be a lot more discerning about what foods I was buying and I came to understand that almost everything contained within the aisles were packed with unsavoury and unhealthy ingredients.

The saying, *"Stick to the perimeter and avoid the aisles,"* is absolutely true. The perimeter of the supermarket is where you will find all your fresh, nutrient-dense foods. The aisles are where you find boxes and packages of junk.

Marketing tactics are so clever these days that we really have no idea what we're eating. Often the wording and packaging are designed to make us believe that what we're buying is good for us.

Take bottled sports water, for example. Next time you're at the supermarket, take a look at some of the ingredients in these drinks. You'll see words like propylene, corn syrup, sucralose, acesulfame K and a series of numbers and letters.

Do these ingredients sound natural or healthy?

Your best bet is to avoid them completely. Some bottled waters have over 30g of sugar per bottle. It's not uncommon for food and beverage companies to breach advertising standards by using words such as 'nutritious' and 'natural' when in fact those products are anything but.

It's also very common for words to be used on packaging that are specifically designed to mislead the consumer. For example, additives can be referred to as 'food processing agents' and MSG is labelled as 621 or 'natural flavouring.'

Nobody really understands what these words mean and we trust that if these foods are available for public consumption, they must be okay, right? Unfortunately, no.

"The food industry is still behaving very badly, producing and marketing unhealthy foods to children in unpardonable amounts. Their pledges to change have amounted to very little. They've shown again and again that they cannot police themselves."

(Kelly Brownell, Director, Rudd Centre for Food Policy and Obesity, Yale University, USA, 2013)

If we really want to understand what we're eating, we must get educated on food labels. The International Numbering System for Food Additives (INS) is accessible online. This is a European-based naming system for food additives, aimed at providing a short designation for what may be a lengthy actual name.

Use this guide the next time you go shopping. We bet you will be shocked at what you find and will start thinking more carefully about what goes in your trolley.

We know that what we've discussed here might be an eye opener and some of it might be hard to take in. You might be thinking, *"But if these things are so bad for us, why are we led to believe otherwise?"*

This is particularly true for meat and dairy products, especially in a country like New Zealand where these industries make up a significant part of our economy. Well, there's part of the answer.

Remember, concern for profits will always over-ride concern for health and this is why we must be aware of what's going on beneath the surface.

There is a minefield of politics and corruption in the food industry and that's a subject for another book, but in the meantime it's up to the individual to become aware of the clever marketing tactics and mistruths being directed our way.

You may be feeling that changing the way you and your family eat is too difficult and be tempted to put it in the too-hard basket. That's entirely your choice but continuing to eat problematic foods that are harming you is a sure way to end up old and sick before your time.

We want to reassure you that the most important thing is progress, not perfection.

No-one is expecting you to change a lifetime of habits overnight – although if you are chronically ill, your motivation to do so and your chances of healing will be much higher.

Start by making some small, gradual changes, such as replacing regular milk with a plant-based milk in your coffee. You will be surprised at how quickly your taste buds change. Or experiment with some plant-based meals and have those one or two nights each week. You could set yourself a goal to cut down on the amount of coffee or alcohol you drink or try going gluten-free.

Doing everything at once can be overwhelming, but it is possible. We give our clients meal plans, grocery lists and recipes to make the whole process super easy and within a couple of weeks, they have made a commitment to themselves that they will never go back to how they were eating before.

We always make sure to offer a cheat meal each week to address any cravings or feelings of deprivation, but it's very common for these cheat meals to become a thing of the past quite quickly because the side effects are too unpleasant!

Nailing your nutrition is one of the absolute best things you will ever do for your health and your happiness. Trust us.

The 10 Leading Causes of Death:

1. *Heart disease**
2. *Cancer**
3. *Accidents*
4. *Chronic Lower Respiratory**
5. *Stroke**
6. *Alzheimer's disease**
7. *Diabetes**
8. *Influenza and Pneumonia*
9. *Kidney disease**
10. *Suicide*

*Related to nutrition

CHAPTER SIX

ENLIGHTENED EXERCISE

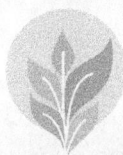

There's no disputing that exercise is good for us and an essential piece of the health puzzle. Most of us are fairly familiar with the benefits of regular exercise, so we are not going to talk about something we already know.

You might be very surprised by what we are about to reveal and it certainly goes against the grain of what most professionals in the fitness industry will tell you. You'd be forgiven for believing everything the professionals say, but the fact is, a lot of the messaging coming from within the industry is misguided and damaging.

It's imperative that you know what type of exercise will allow the body to heal and allow you to experience great overall health. We must also get to the bottom of what messages society is sending us when it comes to exercise and how we can step away from the hype.

Many people come to us and say, *"I'm doing all the right things, but I can't lose weight. I eat really well and work out six times a week but the weight just won't shift."*

These people are exhausting themselves at the gym, because they think that's what they have to do to lose weight. What they don't realise is that their choice of exercise is actually pulling them away from wellness and towards illness.

We need to be educated on the messaging coming from the fitness industry so we can make the right decisions for ourselves, because there's a high chance that the gym you belong to is doing you a great disservice.

We need to get clear on what type of exercise we should be doing and why. The last thing we want for you is to be stuck on an endless merry-go-round of thinking you're doing everything right but getting nowhere. This is not only damaging to your health, it can also be soul-destroying when you don't understand why the changes you wish for aren't happening.

In this chapter, we are able to speak with authority on the subject of exercise because of Steve's strong background in the fitness industry and the thousands of clients he has coached. We are going to discuss the misinformation coming from the fitness industry and how it's contributing to the global health crisis, the very real phenomenon of over-exercising, what exercise you should be doing for your state of health right now and the way in which social media is contributing to misinformation around exercise.

The Problem with the Fitness Industry

It seems like every week there is a new gym opening up somewhere in the area. It promises shiny new facilities, state-of-the-art equipment, lovely bathrooms and saunas, experienced staff and the newest high-impact fitness classes, all for the low price of around $30 per week.

It all sounds exciting, and because we are human, we are naturally drawn to the next new shiny thing to solve all our problems and help us lose that stubborn 10kgs. Of course, there is nothing wrong with a beautiful new fitness centre with an exciting line-up of equipment or fitness classes – if you're 25 and healthy.

If you've been around for a couple more decades than that and you're either on the cusp of chronic illness or right in the thick of it, or even if you're just feeling super stressed, high-impact and high-intensity exercise is the last thing you should be doing. This type of exercise will place excessive stress on an already stressed body. It's something we see time and time again with our clients.

Unfortunately, your average personal trainer at the gym probably won't be aware of this because they are entrenched in an industry that perpetuates the myth that high-intensity exercise is the only real way to get results.

We'll give you an example of one of our real-life clients.

47-year-old Melanie came to see us for the first time. She scored 52 on her adrenal stress quiz, which puts her in the 'crashed zone' for adrenal function. She has a list of symptoms she is battling every single day, including stomach pain and bloating, anxiety, brain fog, hot flushes, joint pain and very low energy levels. She's a wife, a mum of two teenagers, has a stressful full-time job, a mortgage and her husband and kids don't do their fair share around the house. Her spare time is spent running her kids to sports training, checking up on her elderly parents, or catching up on never-ending chores at home.

Because she has so much on her plate, she feels overwhelmed a lot of the time and therefore her body is in 'survival mode' and is constantly pumping adrenaline and cortisol (stress hormones) through her body. This leads to poor sleep and Melanie waking up each morning feeling like she's been run over by a bus. Her first priority each morning is a double shot espresso to help her function, followed by another at 10am.

After a full and busy day at work, she goes to the gym to fit in a Pump class because she's desperate to lose that stubborn body fat around her middle and feels guilty because she hasn't exercised for four days. Then it's home to cook dinner, where she opens a bottle of wine for a glass or two to take the edge off. She's had a hell of a day and she deserves it!

Then it's time to clean up the dinner mess and flop on the couch with a packet of Tim Tams to watch Netflix. She doesn't understand that her low-carbohydrate diet is leading to insatiable cravings late at night. She stays up later than her husband and kids because she needs some 'me time', then finally at around 11.30pm she falls into bed for a fitful and unrefreshing sleep. Wash, rinse, repeat the following day and the day after that.

Melanie is completely overwhelmed and barely coping with life. Her body is so stressed and is desperately trying to tell her to slow down via her numerous symptoms. She's not listening though, brushing them off as minor niggles and part of the normal ageing process.

Each time Melanie goes to the gym, it takes her about four days to recover. She is starting to get more injuries and rather than give her energy, her workouts are completely wiping her out. She thinks she's being lazy because she's not doing enough exercise and perhaps if she did more, she could lose that weight.

What Melanie really needs to do is stop exercising and give her body a break. Her body is crying out to her in distress and she's completely ignoring it. What happens when the body's signals are ignored for a period of time? It decides that enough is enough, and in an effort to slow you down and protect you, pulls on the handbrake in the form of a stroke, heart attack, breakdown, autoimmune disease or something equally devastating.

Rest and recovery is Melanie's absolute priority when she is at the crashed level.

The worrying thing about all this, is that the fitness instructors at Melanie's gym are not aware that her adrenal system has crashed. They have no way of knowing this unless they are actively testing each new client who comes in. Their focus is on securing their portion of Melanie's $30 payment per week, then putting her through her paces with an exercise programme designed to help her 'get fit and lose weight.'

They are not considering the fact that Melanie's body has been under a high level of stress for a period of time and actually needs rest and recovery more than it needs burpees and bicep curls.

This example of Melanie is occurring all over the world. While fitness professionals are trained in exercise techniques and body anatomy and undoubtedly have the desire to help people reach their health and fitness goals, unless they are aware of an individual's sleep and stress levels, they will not be providing the correct level of care for each client.

Just because we see young and fit people in their 20s and 30s getting great results from high intensity exercise, we must remember that their life situation is most likely vastly different from someone in their 40s, 50s and beyond.

For a start, their bodies are younger and have not yet accumulated the wear, tear and abuse that older bodies have. They also may not yet have the same responsibilities and associated stress. We shouldn't expect that a 50-year-old body can cope with the same level of exercise that a 25-year-old can cope with. And this is where the fitness industry is letting us down; through their lack of understanding and knowledge in this area.

Our clients often have interesting stories to share about their experience inside a gym. Lack of personal support is a common theme – as is male trainers directing all their attention to the young ladies in the room and forgetting about everyone else! Another common issue is recurring injury due to over-exercise and lack of recovery time. The problem with a lot of gyms (not all) is that they tend to have a one-size-fits-all approach to health and fitness. This is a mistake and can be problematic if a client has underlying health issues.

The first thing we do when we see a new client for the first time is to assess where they are sitting on the adrenal stress spectrum and from here, we tailor our programmes to suit that individual and their needs. For someone like Melanie who is highly stressed and overwhelmed, we ask them to STOP exercising altogether.

Anything aside from a gentle walk or yoga class is off limits. This is because we understand that high intensity exercise creates more stress for an already stressed body and will push them further into adrenal fatigue and closer to chronic illness.

Don't buy into the misguided theory that High Intensity Interval Training (HIIT) will deliver you the best results. Listen to your body and what it is telling you. If you are constantly sore, fatigued, feeling low or that the next exercise class is another chore to tick off the to-do list, it's time to reassess your exercise habits. It's likely that the best thing you can do right now is rest.

HIIT isn't the only problem. When somebody is stressed, one of the worst things they can do is activate the pectoral muscles at the front of the body or those that move your head forward, such as sit ups or stomach crunches. These are the muscles that automatically get switched on when a dangerous situation pops up suddenly that you need to escape from and your body goes into 'fight or flight' mode.

Instead, concentrate on working the muscles between your shoulder blades and stretching the muscles at the front of your chest, for example, through back extensions or using a rowing machine.

You may have also noticed that our society has also become obsessed with counting calories. There is much hype around 'calories in vs calories out' and everyone is keen to know the calorie breakdown of what they're eating.

Heart rate monitors are also very fashionable and people like to see how many calories they are burning. The danger with this approach is that it perpetuates the myth that weight loss is all about calorie expenditure. We know that this is true to an extent, but there's so much more to weight loss than just calories.

The Right Type of Exercise

Now that we've established that HIIT isn't the best form of exercise if you have a lot of stress in your life, let's talk about the right kind of fitness for you.

If you're in top physical shape, you can do anything you like! Triathlons, ultra-marathons, body building; go for gold! You'll know if you're thriving with great health. You will feel great most of the time, you will be sleeping well, eating well and feeling positive and alive mentally.

If you feel relatively well most of the time, you can do high-impact exercise, but do take note of how you feel afterwards. Exercise should give you pep and energy, so if you start to feel wiped out or struggle to recover, you may need to back off in terms of intensity or frequency.

If you're not in good shape physically, mentally or emotionally, ultra-marathons are not for you and even if you think they could be, you'll likely end up burnt out or with an injury.

Yes, exercise is very important and we would never say that it's not. However, if you are like Melanie and feel overwhelmed and are barely coping, the best thing you can do for yourself right now is focus on rest and recovery. This means having a bath and winding down with a book instead of doing a strenuous workout.

Resting will signal to your body that it's safe and that it can take a break from constantly pumping out adrenaline. When it feels safe, it will start to release body fat. This is why when we tell our stressed clients to stop exercising, they start to see immediate weight loss, much to their surprise.

There is so much conditioning around working out hard to get results that there may need to be a shift in your mindset to give yourself permission to rest. A lot of women in particular struggle with this concept because they're used to a little voice in the back of their head telling them they mustn't be lazy. This isn't about laziness; it's about creating the right environment for your body to heal.

Give yourself permission to back off the exercise and relax and if you struggle with that, remind yourself that your health coach says you must!

If you feel up to it, you can go for a gentle walk around the block, or do some light yoga stretches. Once your body has had the time and space to recover, you can attempt higher-impact exercise. For someone whose adrenal system is at the crashed level, you should allow a recovery period of at least six to eight weeks (sometimes longer), where your first priority is looking after yourself and reducing your workload by up to 50%.

This might sound extreme, but we'll tell you what's more extreme; taking a year or two to recover from a nervous breakdown. You absolutely must give your body the opportunity to rest if you want to get back to feeling your best and prevent further damage to your health.

Social Media

Aspects of social media have also become problematic in the fitness arena. We now have 24/7 access to the highlights reel of everyone else's lives in the form of things like Facebook and Instagram posts. We get sucked into the addiction of scrolling through endless photos of glorious fit, toned and sun-kissed bodies, then left to deal with the aftermath of depression at our own perceived failings in the form of bat-wing arms and wobbly bellies.

While we are aware these images are usually photoshopped or filtered, subconsciously our brains are comparing our perceived less-than-perfect selves to these more-than-perfect others. This is very damaging to mental health and self-esteem and it's not just the younger generation that we need to be worried about. There are plenty of middle-aged and elderly people feeling miserable about themselves after comparing themselves to their photoshopped peers.

A big problem with exposure to these types of images is that they reinforce the false and detrimental message that skinny equals happy. Society has a ridiculous obsession with lean and fat-free bodies, particularly for women, and we're seeing more examples of women busting their backsides to get a six-pack.

For a woman, a six-pack is very difficult to achieve and takes a lot of dedicated hard work and discipline. Female bodies are not designed to be hard and muscular; they are designed to be soft and curvy to support childbirth and nurturing. How we got to a place where six-packs and big biceps on women are celebrated is simply bizarre and unhealthy.

Disclaimer: We're not calling YOU bizarre if you are a female and naturally have a muscular physique or if you have worked hard to get one. We are saying that the hell-bent obsession for women who are not naturally muscular to get this way, is not a healthy way to live.

Even though we live in a society that values beauty over all else, we don't have to buy into it. If you feel like your self-esteem is taking a hit every time you see something on social media that makes you feel yuck about yourself, choose to step away and create personal boundaries around what you are accepting into your life. It takes strength to do this for sure and it can be a daily practice to remind yourself that you don't subscribe to this false and shallow belief system.

It sounds like a cliché, but finding happiness and contentment does not automatically happen when you lose that excess body fat. We've had clients who have shed heaps of weight, but still have underlying stress that hasn't miraculously disappeared with the weight. Yes, it goes without saying that losing excess weight will do wonders for your health and you will no doubt feel more confident, but it's not the magic fix for everything.

In our personal experience, health and happiness go hand in hand and it's impossible to have one without the other. If finding happiness is your ultimate goal, start by taking care of your health first.

For some of you, reassessing the way you exercise will be challenging because your identity may be tied up in being 'fit and healthy' and you are conditioned to the mindset that hard exercise is best. We encourage you to actively work on changing your beliefs around exercise if you are currently struggling with any area of your health and wellbeing, because not doing so is likely to be detrimental in the long term.

Please rest assured that you don't need to give up exercising forever; this is more of a temporary break to get your physical and mental self to a point where it can handle the exercise you enjoy. Once you take the hard workouts off your plate and replace them with either a gentle walk (or a hot bath!) and notice your body starting to recover, you will probably appreciate the break and realise it's the best thing you could have done.

You may have a current gym membership that you don't want to go to waste, so ask if you can put it on hold for a couple of months or transfer it to someone else who can use it. Most gyms are fairly accommodating in this regard but don't be surprised if they look at you blankly when you explain the reason! And don't let anyone else's opinion of what you are choosing to do sway you. Your personal trainer or jogging buddies might not understand or try to talk you out of it but be confident in your decision and know it's the best thing for your health right now.

If you are someone who exercises hard or puts a lot of pressure on yourself to exercise, you may need to be honest and check whether you have unrealistic or unhealthy expectations around body image. If the answer is yes, we suggest you reduce or eliminate your exposure to the types of things that are perpetuating these feelings.

Take a break from Instagram or that Facebook page for fitness junkies. While these tools masquerade as a source of entertainment or useful information, they could be subconsciously affecting your self-esteem and perception of who you should be or what you should look like.

Another thing we must mention is that you can never out-run or out-exercise a deeper emotional problem, even if you feel like exercise is your form of stress relief. We've seen many clients who have problems going on at home or work, and over-exercising is their way of dealing with them. One likely outcome of this is an exercise addiction.

No amount of exercise can resolve the root cause of a problem, yet the elusive chase continues, leading to more and more exercise in an attempt to feel better. They think, *"Perhaps if I get super lean and super fit, I can be happy."*

You may end up with a body to die for, but you'll never be truly happy if you don't resolve the root cause of the underlying stress. Another likely outcome is burnout, where the adrenal system can't cope with the amount of adrenaline required to keep the body functioning at such a high level.

If you're feeling less than healthy and energetic, do yourself a favour and lay off the intense exercise. It will be one of the most important things you do on your road to recovery.

CHAPTER SEVEN

GUTS AND GLORY

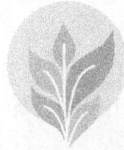

What really happens when food travels down the throat and into the stomach is still a bit of a mystery. The whole digestive system is made up of incredible intricacies that are difficult to comprehend and digestion is one of least understood aspects of human physiology. We believe that if it was better understood, the medical community would stop denying the fundamental importance of nutrition as a means of caring for and healing the body.

On a positive note, there is a lot of research going on right now about the importance of a healthy microbiome. The microbiome are the bacteria, viruses and yeasts that populate the gut and is now accepted as an essential part of our overall health. Not only does it help to digest food, it's also in charge of regulating metabolism and blood sugar, manufacturing vitamins and influencing brain chemistry and genetic expression.

"Treat our microbiome like a garden – we need to nourish the soil (intestines) for healthy plants (bacteria), while minimising weeds (disease-causing microbes.)"

(Tim Spector, Professor of Genetic Epidemiology)

Understanding the significant influence of the gut on our health and wellbeing is crucial if we want to address any symptoms or conditions going on in the body. We must be clear on the factors that are contributing to poor gut health and how to overcome them if we want to experience optimal health.

Conventional medicine is missing a crucial link between the state of the gut and mental health, and it's fundamental that we understand that link so we can start treating mental health issues more effectively. We must also be aware of the types of fads and trends we need to steer clear of if we want to avoid draining our wallets and being left with nothing to show for it.

It's quite worrying how many clients come to us because they are experiencing problems in the gut area. Gas, bloating, constipation, diarrhoea, cramps and severe pain are all signs that something in the gut and digestive system isn't working correctly.

Many of these clients are given diagnoses such as Crohn's disease, colitis, diverticulitis or Irritable Bowel Syndrome (IBS) and are told nothing much can be done and they must take medication to help with the symptoms. Much of the time, this is absolute rubbish. Simple lifestyle changes that focus on healing the gut can often completely reverse these unpleasant symptoms and allow for a very normal and pain-free life.

The consequences of not fully understanding the role of the gut in our health is dire, because those who are suffering will never be able to get to the root cause of the issue nor will they know how to fix it. This is especially devastating for those who suffer from any kind of mental illness.

Right now, they are being fobbed off by doctors with packets of anti-depressant or anti-anxiety medication, when in reality there is a relatively straightforward solution. Think about how many lives could be saved from suicide if the gut-brain connection was better understood. When we don't understand the true causes of a sick gut and how to remedy it, we risk being sucked into gimmicky fads that do nothing beneficial and can even be quite damaging.

Below we are going to discuss why gut health is so important, the factors that create poor gut health, how to restore a healthy gut, why this is so important for mental health and the fads and trends to steer well clear of.

The Guts of the Gut

The gut is made up of the stomach, small intestine, large intestine (which includes the colon), liver and gallbladder. It's also responsible for the break down, digestion and absorption of nutrients, expelling toxins and waste and maintaining a strong immune system. Various pathogens such as mould, fungus, worms and viruses can infiltrate the gut and can create a breeding ground for all sorts of illnesses. It's really important to know how to prevent this from happening and how to deal with it if it does.

Phrases such as 'gut instinct', or 'feeling gutted' or 'that must have taken guts to do' indicate that we do understand on an instinctual level the importance of the gut. Our emotions are also strongly linked to the gut. Think about when a stressful situation arises, and how you feel in your gut.

If you receive some emotionally distressing news, you may feel like your gut shuts down, where you get a churning, sick feeling and are unable to eat. This is because our emotions determine whether our gut functions calmly or in a state of turmoil. Your gut can't deal with stressful emotions and digest food at the same time.

Let's take a look at some of the main causes or poor gut health.

Leaky Gut Syndrome

Leaky gut syndrome, also known as intestinal permeability is a condition where ulcers, bacteria or superbugs can cause breakages in the lining of the gastrointestinal tract and allow pathogens and intestinal matter to leach into the bloodstream. Another cause can be when the colon is punctured during a colonoscopy.

An alternative view of the cause of leaky gut has also come to light in the past few years called ammonia permeability and is related to hydrochloric acid levels in the gut. Hydrochloric acid is a stomach acid that helps the body to break down, digest and absorb nutrients such as protein, while also eliminating bacteria and viruses in the stomach.

If hydrochloric acid levels become too low, food won't be sufficiently digested and will instead lie in the intestines and rot (putrefy). Putrefaction can create a toxic gas, resulting in symptoms such as digestive discomfort, bloating and chronic dehydration – or sometimes no symptoms at all.

Eventually over time, hydrochloric acid can diminish in the stomach and bad acids can take its place. These bad acids travel up the oesophagus, causing symptoms such as acid reflux. The gut lining also starts to create mucus to protect you from the bad acids. If you are getting a lot of mucus in your throat for no apparent reason, it's likely that the bad acids are eating away at your stomach and oesophagus lining, resulting in your body producing mucus to keep you safe. Mucus can also be produced if you eat a lot of dairy products, because these foods encourage pathogenic and viral growth in the body.

The toxic gas produced from decomposing food in your intestinal tract is able to float into the bloodstream and this is what is known as ammonia permeability. This gas floats around the liver, gallbladder, bloodstream and intestinal tract and it is this gas that creates a lot of the symptoms associated with leaky gut syndrome.

While this information is very alternative and not found within the conventional medical field, we have taken this approach on board when dealing with the gut health of our clients and have found it to be very accurate. Once hydrochloric acid is restored in the stomach, food is able to be properly broken down and absorbed and waste is able to move through the body freely, completely eliminating the putrefaction process described above. Once the elimination pathways are cleared, healing can start to happen at a rapid pace.

Toxic Heavy Metals

With our modern lifestyles, it is almost impossible not to ingest toxic heavy metals such as mercury, aluminium, nickel, arsenic and lead. Ingestion can occur through industrial exposure, foods, medicines, air or water pollution, improperly coated food containers or cookware, or the ingestion of lead-based paints.

These heavy metals are literally heavy and they sink into your intestinal tract and accumulate in the liver, gallbladder and brain. Not only are they poisonous to the body, they also feed bacteria, fungi, viruses, parasites and worms, which then release toxic gases when they consume the heavy metals.

Vitamin B12 Deficiency

Conventional medicine would have us believe that we gain Vitamin B12 through the consumption of meat. If this was true, meat-eaters wouldn't be deficient in this vitamin. The reality is, almost everyone has a Vitamin B12 deficiency and it's a myth that meat-eaters are immune.

Vitamin B12 is actually abundant on the leaves of leafy greens and these are the best source, but we should also use a Vitamin B12 supplement. Vitamin B12 production and availability start to plummet when there is low hydrochloric acid, heavy metal toxicity and ammonia permeability happening in the gut. Even if blood tests show you have an adequate supply of B12, it doesn't mean this precious vitamin is being absorbed or utilised by the central nervous system. Lack of B12 is a very real deficiency with serious health consequences.

The Problem with Gluten

We've already talked briefly about gluten in the nutrition chapter, but we want to give you more background about why it can be so problematic. Even if you don't think you have a problem with gluten, you probably do. You might not be experiencing symptoms of gluten sensitivity, but it may still be damaging the lining of your gut, leading to leaky gut syndrome.

Gluten sensitivity seems to be getting worse among the general population and many people now are going gluten-free and noticing how much better they feel without it. Gluten content in grains has increased over the years, which makes digestion more difficult.

Research over a 30-year-period by Dr Tom O'Bryan has also shown that many autoimmune conditions have their roots in gluten consumption. This claim will likely be rubbished by your GP, because once again the importance of nutrition is not recognised by conventional medicine.

We take all of our clients off gluten and without fail their gut and digestive problems disappear very, very quickly. Removing gluten from the diet is a particularly important piece of the puzzle for people suffering autoimmune dysfunction in the gut area. We have seen many instances of clients who have been able to reverse their symptoms when gluten is removed.

Our client Jenny came to us feeling absolutely miserable because she was suffering from constant tummy pain, bloating and constipation. These symptoms had been bothering her for years, but after several routine doctors' tests she was told there was nothing wrong and nothing could be done.

Understandably, Jenny was at her wits end and the pain was affecting her mental health. She felt very low, depressed and frustrated that she was unable to find a solution to the pain and discomfort.

Within one week of following our meal plans and removing gluten, her tummy pain had reduced by 80% and within two weeks, not only had the pain disappeared completely, but she was also now having regular bowel motions with no sign of constipation.

The Gut's Link to Mental Health

Another area that is still not widely understood within conventional medicine is that gut health is very strongly linked to mental health. This is because up to 90% of our serotonin (happy hormone) is produced in the gut. Also, for each signal the brain sends to the gut, the gut sends nine signals back to the brain. If the gut is in a state of distress due to an over-abundance of unhealthy gut bacteria, we can expect our mental health to be less than ideal.

It is very common for our clients to be experiencing an array of mental health issues when they first come to see us, such as depression, anxiety, brain fog, memory loss, concentration problems, migraines and headaches. When we put them onto a healthy food plan and start replenishing the gut with plenty of beneficial gut bacteria, their mental health starts to rapidly improve. Brain fog and memory and concentration issues evaporate and depression and anxiety significantly lessen or disappear altogether.

Restoring Gut Health

Gut health can be restored by focusing on restoring hydrochloric acid in the stomach, reducing heavy metal toxicity, addressing ammonia permeability, ensuring an adequate supply of Vitamin B12 and removing gluten from the diet.

Restoring hydrochloric acid can be achieved by removing the foods that strip the stomach of this essential acid. These 'trouble-makers' are listed in the Nutrition chapter. Excess meat in the diet also strips the hydrochloric acid from the stomach, which is why high fat trends like the Keto diet should be treated with caution.

The best way to restore hydrochloric acid is through a diet of fresh, nutrient-dense whole foods. When this acid is restored, ammonia permeability is reduced because the acid helps break down and digest food correctly, rather than allowing undigested food to putrefy in the digestive tract.

Toxic heavy metals can lead to multiple problems if not addressed, but they can be relatively easy to remove from the gut. If you have any kind of gut illness, it's safe to assume that part of the problem can be attributed to heavy metal toxicity. Removing heavy metals from the gut can be achieved by eliminating foods such as tuna and reducing your exposure to the things mentioned under 'toxic heavy metals' above.

While plenty of leafy greens are important for Vitamin B12, everyone should take a Vitamin B12 supplement to ensure they are getting an adequate supply. Look for Vitamin B12 in spray or dropper form, which is more easily absorbed by the body than a capsule or tablet. Make sure you check the label and avoid unnecessary ingredients. The best form of B12 should contain methylcobalamin as the sole ingredient.

Removing gluten from the diet is also an important step in restoring the health of your gut. Remember, gluten appears in foods you least expect, so be sure to read food labels carefully.

Beware of Synthetic Probiotics

Probiotics in capsule form are all the rage these days, but let's be clear on what you're actually getting when you're spending your hard-earned cash. There is absolutely no evidence to show that cultured probiotics sitting on the shelves of a health food store or fermented foods claiming to have beneficial bacteria are actually entering your gut and performing the way they are expected to.

In fact, we don't endorse taking probiotics in pill form because there is a well-founded theory that by the time they transition from the shelf to your gut, the beneficial bacteria are already dead. Also, factory produced probiotics never even get to the part of the small intestine that needs them the most.

Trends and marketing hype are largely behind the sale of probiotics. Buyer beware.

There are however probiotics that do stay alive inside the gut and can restore intestinal flora. These special probiotics live on leafy greens, fruits, wild foods, herbs and vegetables and garner energy from the sun. Not only do they restore the precious beneficial bacteria our guts so desperately need, they also create a form of Vitamin B12 that the body most recognises.

You can get a fantastic supply of probiotics from sprouts such as kale, sunflower, alfalfa, broccoli, clover, fenugreek, lentils and mustard seeds. The best way to get probiotics into your gut is by eating leafy greens straight from your garden, unscrubbed (unless they are really dirty) and uncooked, because millions of amazing probiotics exist on their surface. Be sure to only follow this method when you know the vegetables haven't been sprayed or contaminated with toxins that could make you sick.

Growing your own sprouts or herbs inside or outside is another great form of probiotics. All these forms of probiotics have an incredible effect on the digestive and immune systems. The key thing to remember is to try and eat as many probiotics on living fruits, vegetables, herbs, wild foods and leafy greens as you can, because they will support the environment of the entire gut.

In order to restore gut health, you must also be aware of the things that kill off the beneficial gut bacteria and try to avoid them as much as possible. These include caffeine, alcohol, sugar, food sensitivities, stress hormones and some anti-inflammatory steroid medications. When you think about how often we are exposing ourselves to these trouble-makers, it's no surprise that so many people have problems with their gut and therefore overall state of health.

You can't have a festering mess of a gut and expect to be healthy.

Fads and Trends

Fads, trends, tricks, gimmicks, whatever you want to call them, are rife in both the conventional and alternative medical fields. When you are desperately unwell, it's very natural to be drawn into these trends in the hope of finding the magic remedy you're searching for. Most of the time though, they are all about fancy and clever marketing strategies and profits and very little about your health.

There are so many fads on the market related to gut health, but here are some of the most common ones to be aware of and treat with caution.

Fermented Foods

Back in the old days, fermentation was used by almost every culture for foods such as fruits, vegetables and dairy products for the sole purpose of survival. There was no such thing as refrigeration or a supermarket just around the corner.

These days there's the belief that because fermentation helped our ancestors survive, they are healthy. When you start to drill down into what is actually happening during the fermentation process however, you start to realise it's not all it's cracked up to be.

Thousands of years ago, fermentation was more about preventing starvation than actually delivering any real health benefits.

The bacteria in fermented foods thrive off the decay process and are similar to bacteria that start to decompose rotting flesh. They are a very different bacteria from the beneficial bacteria we need in our gut. Probiotics on fresh fruits, vegetables, leafy greens, wild foods and herbs are restorative in the gut and have a potent power that the bacteria in fermented food just don't have.

The bacteria in foods like sauerkraut, salami, soy sauce and kombucha are useless for your gut. In most people, they are harmless and expelled through the digestive tract and eating a little of these foods won't do any serious damage. For some people it's a different story, however. The body can perceive these bacteria as invaders and will launch an attack to expel them. This can result in unpleasant symptoms such as nausea, gas, bloating, pain and diarrhoea. Most of the time the symptoms are temporary and resolve once the bacteria is out of the body.

If you really love fermented foods and they don't do you any harm, it's fine to consume them in moderate quantities, but just be aware they aren't doing anything beneficial for your gut.

We've also been led down the garden path when it comes to probiotic yoghurt. Yoghurt is the last thing you should be eating if you are chronically unwell, because viral and pathogenic activity in the body regard dairy as a fuel source and start to thrive, replicate and defecate in the body – gross!

Not only that, if the yoghurt has been pasteurised (treated with mild heat), the probiotics have been killed anyway. Beneficial probiotics that do survive in raw yoghurt cannot withstand natural acids in the stomach and won't reach the intestinal tract, where they are needed the most. Also, if your gut is unhappy with an abundance of unproductive gut bacteria, the beneficial probiotics will not over-ride the problems that these bad bacteria create.

Baking Soda and Candida

Candida is very often misunderstood as a trouble-maker in the gut, whereas it's actually the *symptom* of an unhappy gut. When your gut is dysfunctional as a result of things like toxic heavy metals and other toxins lurking around inside, pathogenic infections can be the result.

The theory that baking soda is a cure for candida is misguided. This 'remedy' for stomach discomfort has been around for a long time. In fact, I can remember my grandmother mixing baking soda with water on a daily basis to help with acid reflux.

All baking soda does is act as an abrasive inside the gut and create an imbalance. Large doses of baking soda can create a toxic crisis for the body because it's irritating to the stomach and intestinal tract, particularly if that area is already inflamed. This can lead to vomiting, bloating, diarrhoea and other problems. It can also lead to gastric spasms, a worsening of fungal and bacterial infections and a worsening of digestive issues.

Apple Cider Vinegar

Contrary to popular belief, ingesting apple cider vinegar will not help your gut. Not only is it an irritant, it also causes dehydration, wears down tooth enamel, weakens the glands in the stomach and stresses the liver. Any kind of digestive issue will be worsened by apple cider vinegar and it's likely you will end up with additional bloating.

If you read the 'Restoring Gut Health' section and feel that the steps required to create a healthy gut is a difficult and overwhelming task, please be assured that it's not. We understand that changing the way you have eaten for many years can be daunting, but it's actually very straightforward when you know what to do. Our clients are pleasantly surprised when we give them meal plans and recipes and they realise how easy it is.

You may be afraid of missing out on all the things you love to eat, but we can assure you that when you start fuelling your body with the fresh, nutrient-dense foods it needs, your taste and desire for all those things will rapidly diminish.

Also, your gut will be so happy and functioning so well that it's very unlikely you will want to go back to eating all those trouble-makers, because the side effects just aren't worth it. Of all our hundreds and hundreds of clients, we can't recall a single one who willingly goes back to their past eating habits once we show them healthier alternatives.

We are very lucky these days to be surrounded by an abundance of alternative foods such as gluten-free products and plant-based milks, which makes cooking delicious and nutritious meals a breeze.

Resist overcomplicating things or get trapped by a this-is-too-hard mindset. If you want to experience vibrant health and wellbeing, it all starts in the gut.

CHAPTER EIGHT

SUPERIOR SLEEP

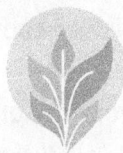

Human beings have evolved to need plenty of sleep, and if you don't sleep properly or don't get enough, everything else starts to fall apart. Lack of sleep can result in serious long-term complications for the body.

We have come to realise that sleep is the most understated and under-coached cornerstone of the health industry and this is where our coaching programmes really start to shine. We put a lot of emphasis on sleep because we understand that it is the foundation for every part of health and wellbeing.

A lack of understanding around the reasons for poor sleep is problematic because it becomes very difficult for people to overcome sleep issues if they don't know what is causing them in the first place.

We tend to think that lack of sleep just makes you tired the next day, but the impacts of long-term sleep problems are significant and serious. It is easy to write sleep off as not a 'big deal' – especially when it comes to healing the body – but in actual fact, it is crucial.

If you want optimal health and wellbeing, you need to learn how to sleep properly and relying on sleeping pills from your doctor will never teach you how to do that. Sleeping pills are a temporary solution for those times you absolutely must sleep but should not be treated as a long-term solution. If you've ever relied on sleeping pills then battled chronic insomnia when you try to come off them, you'll know that sleeping pills can cause more harm than good.

We always ask our clients about the quality of their sleep. Usually, the answer is something like, *"Oh, I sleep pretty well. I go to bed at 10pm and wake up at 6am so I get a full eight hours."*

We then ask if they wake up feeling refreshed in the morning. 90% of the time, the answer is no.

This is an indicator that their sleep is not as deep and restful as they think.

You might be surprised at how many people struggle to sleep. Perhaps you aren't surprised, because you're one of them! Sleep difficulties are not something that magically improve with age, so unless you get to the root cause of the issues now, you risk an ongoing battle with sleep into the future and the associated health risks.

You will also most likely be told by your doctor that lack of sleep is due to things like anger, grief, depression, worry or pain. These might be very real reasons, but there's so much more to understand that isn't acknowledged by conventional medicine.

We are going to teach you the main reasons behind poor sleep, the consequences of poor sleep and how you can experience the deep, blissful, restful sleep your body craves and deserves.

Sleep disorders come in many different forms. You may be someone who can fall asleep straight away, but you wake up too early in the morning. Perhaps you wake in the middle of the night and lie there for hours, before dropping off again just before it's time to get up. Perhaps you toss and turn all night and wake up feeling exhausted. Maybe you sink into a deep sleep and then wake up with jerky movements from an arm or leg.

Below we will look at some of the main reasons for these sleep disorders:

A Poor Lifestyle

The first is a poor lifestyle, where high levels of stress lead to poor sleep, which leads to drinking too much coffee to keep you awake, which leads to high stress and so the cycle repeats. You get stuck on a merry-go-round and this leads to stubborn body fat, among several other problems.

Modern lifestyles have a lot to answer for when it comes to sleep, or lack of. Generally speaking, people are sleeping a lot less now than what their ancestors did. Longer working hours, shift work and the pressures of being constantly available via smart phones mean we are generally getting to bed later than we should be.

Digestive Issues

As we've already discussed, the gut-brain connection is very strong. If there are any issues going on inside your gut, such as bloating, digestive pain or cramping, these are directly communicated to the brain, which can then trigger the nervous system and keep you alert.

When someone is highly stressed, the excess adrenaline in the body can inflame the gut and when food passes through the intestines, it activates the nerves that connect to the brain. Often you can't feel this inflammation and you wonder why on earth you're wide awake for no apparent reason.

Emotional Issues

Emotional trauma, whether major or minor, can cause physical repercussions in the body. Emotional wounds can burn out the neurological system and create scar tissue on the brain. This can lead to persistent lack of sleep.

Sleep Anxiety

Sleep anxiety can be a result of nightmares, Post Traumatic Stress Disorder (PTSD) or Obsessive Compulsive Disorder (OCD). It can also be caused by neurological disturbances such as nerve sensitivity that can cause anxiety.

Sleep anxiety can also be caused by toxic heavy metals in the brain, leading to a panic response, restlessness or a feeling of not being able to think straight. As already mentioned, gut problems can also lead to being woken in the middle of the night and can bring with it a feeling of anxiousness for no reason.

A Sick Liver

When you go to sleep at night, your liver sleeps, too. Around 3am – 4am after a good rest, it gets to work by processing all the toxins and gunk in the body, getting them ready to be flushed out with a big glass of water when you wake up in the morning.

If you have a sick, stagnant or sluggish liver due to a diet high in processed foods and excess fats, it can malfunction in the early hours of the morning, resulting in spasms that can wake you up. This can explain why you can fall asleep normally when you first go to bed, wake up in the night, then get back to sleep again. It can also explain those nights when you drift in and out of sleep for the whole night.

Adrenal Fatigue

The words 'fatigue' can be misleading when it comes to sleep. Anyone with ongoing adrenal fatigue will tell you that sleep doesn't come easily just because the body is in a state of fatigue.

Adrenal fatigue is caused by adrenal glands that seesaw between producing too much and too little adrenaline. They can be underactive during the day, leading to a feeling of lethargy, then become overactive at night, thus disturbing sleep.

Sleep Apnoea

Obstructive sleep apnoea can be caused by issues such as inflammation of the bronchial tubes or tonsils, postnasal drip, excess mucus, chronic sinusitis, edema and excess weight putting pressure on the chest and throat. People with this type of sleep apnoea often need special machines to force air through their airways as they sleep. This type of sleep apnoea can be relieved by eating foods that don't create excess mucus and inflammation in the body, such as dairy products.

Non-obstructive sleep apnoea isn't relieved by machines because the issue stems from the neurological system. Toxins such as toxic heavy metals and herbicides create chemical imbalances in the brain, leading to tiny seizures which are enough to create a pause in breath.

Neurological Issues

Serious sleep issues such as insomnia are often caused by neurological distress in the body and dysfunctional adrenal glands. The foundation of this type of sleep disorder is PTSD resulting from a traumatic event.

Whether this event occurred in the distant past or more recently, it can create neurological issues, leading to lack of sleep and involuntary jerking movements. Lack of magnesium is also a factor.

Impacts from Loss of Sleep

Anyone who has ever experienced a sleepless night will know how much of an impact lack of sleep can have. The odd sleepless night here or there is inevitable and no big deal, particularly if there is a direct known cause, such as a teething baby in the household or feelings of worry over a workplace conflict. When the odd sleepless night becomes more regular though, this is far more serious and resembles a unique type of hell. Even lack of sleep over two or three nights can be enough to put immense stress on our physical and mental wellbeing. What is even more distressing is when we don't know the cause of our sleepless nights, which then creates a vicious cycle of worry and even less sleep.

A lack of sleep is a dysfunction in the body, and chronic lack of sleep over the long term has been shown to cause early death. Sleep is so important to allow the body to rest and repair and is essential for the correct function of all our organs.

Sleep is more important for weight loss than exercise. A lack of sleep puts the body into survival mode, and when the body is in this state, it will cling to body fat for dear life. Weight loss without good quality sleep is very difficult to achieve.

The stress response in the body from lack of sleep not only leads to eating more calories, it also contributes to fat deposits around the abdomen, even if you are working hard at the gym. If you are generally healthy and feel like you are eating well and working out hard and are not seeing any weight loss, be honest with yourself about how much sleep you are getting.

Those who sleep only five or six hours per night gain more weight than those who sleep for eight hours. We worked with one young mum who was only sleeping for one hour per night. After sticking with our programme for five weeks, she was getting a full eight hours of sleep. Only then was she able to lose weight.

There is a magic number when it comes to sleep that seems to clearly predict weight gain and poor health and this is seven and a half hours. Most people do best with more and very few do well with less. One way to determine how much sleep is best for you is to think about how much sleep you get when you go away on holiday and don't have to wake up to an alarm – although the first few days may not be an accurate measure because you may be catching up on lost sleep.

Lack of sleep also makes it very hard to recover from a physical workout, and therefore building muscle becomes near impossible. Those who don't sleep enough also have a much higher risk for obesity, diabetes, depression, heart problems and cancer.

One crucial consequence of lack of sleep is that our liver can't carry out its multiple functions correctly overnight. Because the liver is our #1 detox organ, it needs a good eight hours of rest to clean up the body and filter out all the toxins.

Another factor that is not clearly understood is that sleep quality is strongly linked to gut health. As already discussed, 90% of our serotonin (happy hormone) is produced in the gut. From serotonin we produce melatonin, a hormone essential for deep, restful sleep.

There is also a dangerous theory that alcohol can help us sleep better. While drinking alcohol before bed can help you drop off to sleep faster, it worsens REM (rapid eye movement) sleep and therefore can keep you awake during the night for long periods and give you an overall worse quality of sleep.

Restoring Sleep

Restoring deep sleep can take time (weeks or months) because the body needs to cleanse and heal. We have seen many clients who don't sleep properly, including one lady in her 80s who became a chronic insomniac after the death of her husband.

After just a few weeks on our programme, she began sleeping through the night and hasn't looked back. Her whole life has been transformed for the better as a result.

Even though good quality sleep is essential for the body's ability to rest, recover and repair, it's reassuring to know that even when you're not getting enough sleep, your body is still able to heal to some degree.

The body's healing processes are in full force between the hours of 10pm to 2am, so even if you're wide awake during those hours, part of your brain is still asleep and allowing for healing to take place. If you are asleep during those hours, your body undergoes a state of rapid healing.

A Pre-Bed Routine

In our coaching programmes, we recommend a very effective pre-bed routine to help the body wind down and prepare for sleep, which we are going to share with you here. It can take time for your body to re-learn how to sleep correctly and it may take a few weeks before you see a noticeable improvement. Be patient, persevere and trust that your body knows what it's doing.

Also keep in mind that this routine will only be effective if the other four pillars of health are working in harmony. If you have three glasses of wine and Burger King for dinner, or you have a lot of background stress you haven't dealt with, you can't expect to have a great sleep.

- At least one hour after dinner and one hour before bed, drink a cup of chamomile tea. Chamomile is a safe, mild sleep inducer that signals to your body it's time for rest. If you don't like the taste of chamomile on its own, put a peppermint tea bag in the cup to disguise the taste. Alternatively, you can let the tea cool then drink it in one go. There are plenty of chamomile tea blends available now so choose one you like.

- If you have a sweet tooth and find yourself reaching for sweets after dinner, satisfy your craving with one or two pieces of dark chocolate. Make sure you read the label and avoid anything with dairy products. Look for the 80-90% cocoa varieties. Dark chocolate is more satisfying than milk chocolate because it has a slight bitterness, which prevents you wanting to go back for more and more. Have your dark chocolate with your cup of chamomile tea.

- Soak in a hot bath for 20 minutes, three times per week. Make the water as hot as you can stand. If you have blood pressure issues, are pregnant or highly stressed, make sure the water is lukewarm only because your body will be unable to correctly regulate body temperature. Add one cup of Epsom salts for magnesium absorption and a quarter cup of baking soda to calm the central nervous system. This is a great way to unwind before bed – just be sure to lock to the door in case any other little family members decide it's a great time for a chat! If you don't have a bath, soak your feet in a tub instead.

- At least thirty minutes before bed turn off your smartphone, Kindle or iPad. The blue light from these devices stimulates cortisol (alert hormone) and signals to your body it's time to wake up by blocking melatonin. Resist watching television directly before bedtime and we recommend not having a television in the bedroom.

- Lie flat in bed with one pillow beneath your head. This places your body into parasympathetic dominance (rest, digest, repair) and signals to the body that it's safe. It also opens up the rib cage and allows the free flow of oxygen through the body.

- Read a light-hearted book or magazine. Avoid reading anything too stimulating that may activate the brain too much, such as work-related documents or news articles that induce fear or worry. After 15-20 minutes, you will most likely find yourself getting drowsy and ready for sleep.

- Aim for lights out at 10pm at the latest.

More Sleep Remedies

It's a good idea to consider whether the temperature in your bedroom is adversely affecting your sleep; an ideal temperature is around 18°C. Exposure to negative ions can also be beneficial; these are molecules floating in the air that have been charged with electricity and are found in natural settings especially where there is water and vegetation. To get the benefits from negative ions, spend as much time as possible in the fresh air.

Another strategy to help the body prepare for sleep is to write down anything that is on your mind before getting into bed. You can simply do a 'brain dump' or write down any actions you need to take to resolve a problem you are dealing with. When you train yourself to do this regularly, unresolved worries or thoughts will no longer interrupt your sleep time.

Detoxification of the body is a fundamental component of healing sleep issues. Increasing the amount of fresh fruit and vegetables in your diet will raise your immune system and activate the detoxification process. Healing the liver is crucial to allow for correct detoxification.

If you suffer from adrenal fatigue, grazing on several small meals throughout the day is the way to go. This is to ensure your already fatigued adrenal glands don't have to continuously pump out adrenaline when your blood sugar levels drop.

Naps during the day are not just for nanas and children. If you feel you need a daytime nap to recover from a late night or because you are simply feeling like you need it, it's a good idea to have one.

For digestive issues, make sure you are eating plenty of natural probiotics in the form of fresh fruits and vegetables. Supplement your existing diet with fresh, raw and organic produce. Sprouts grown on your benchtop are also amazing forms of probiotics.

If you have sleep apnoea, refer to the list of healing foods below to reduce mucus and inflammation and improve neurological function.

Anxiety sufferers need some TLC via comforting foods such as sweet potatoes or herbal tea with raw honey. Rest assured that anxiety-induced sleep problems are not your fault. There are many underlying reasons for anxiety, as mentioned above. Focus on the foods below to help reduce anxious feelings.

Neurological issues that disrupt sleep can also be eased by focusing on the list of foods below because they help to calm the body and brain, provide antioxidants and cleanse toxins.

Healing Foods for Sleep

The best foods to promote healthy sleep are spinach, celery, asparagus, lettuce, coriander, garlic, wild blueberries, sweet potatoes, cherries, bananas and mangoes.

And remember, it's super important to eat carbohydrates at night to lower cortisol levels and give your body the best chance to fall into a deep restful sleep.

If you have struggled for a long time to get a good night's sleep, you may have developed a mistrust in your body and its ability to sleep well. This is a very real phenomenon in our modern society and many people have just come to accept they can't sleep.

The human body is biologically designed to sleep deeply and restfully every night, but as you've just read, there are several reasons why sleep is elusive for many of us.

Never underestimate the powerful link between nutrition and sleep. If you eat junk food all day and into the evening, you can expect a rubbish sleep. If you fuel your body with the goodness it needs, your gut will behave itself, your hormones will recalibrate and your body will sleep the way nature intended.

It can take time to resolve a sleep issue. It will take time for the body to cleanse itself of toxins, heal and rebuild, so in the meantime, remind yourself that the body is very intelligent and can't forget how to sleep.

It is, in fact, capable of great sleep, given the right environment and support.

CHAPTER NINE

SUSTAINABLE STRESS SOLUTIONS

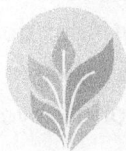

S tress is a word that is thrown around a lot these days. It seems we are all suffering from some kind of stress, from relationship stress to financial stress to work stress. To a large extent, our modern lifestyles have a lot to answer for here. We've got mortgages, relationships, businesses, jobs, kids, interviews and to-do lists. These are all real forms of stress but wait – there's more!

Stress doesn't only relate to being busy and wound up. We've also got food stress, environmental stress, chemical stress, historical and unresolved stress and electronic device stress. Let's not mention pandemic stress! Is reading all that stressing you out? Us too.

As a society, we are more stressed than ever. We hear you saying: *"But, what about people who lived through world wars and depressions and plagues? What about back in the old days when hunters had to run away from lions and bears in the jungle? Surely that was more stressful than the world we live in now?"*

Yes, those events were incredibly stressful for those who had to live through them. The difference between that stress and the type of stress we have now, is that many of us are now living in a state of stress 24/7 for years and years on end and it's wreaking havoc on our health.

Stress is another factor that is often overlooked in the health and wellbeing industry. We all know it exists, but it's not talked about very much. It's unlikely that your doctor, naturopath, personal trainer or nutritionist will take the time to delve into what type of stress you have in your life, or how you are addressing it.

It's important to understand how significant and far-reaching the effects of stress are on both ourselves and the people around us. We must recognise how stress is fuelling and compounding our health issues and the methods we can use to overcome it if we want to experience great health.

We must also acknowledge a form of stress that is being widely overlooked but plays a significant role in our overall state of health and that is feelings of bitterness or resentment towards others.

Approximately 50% of our clients come to us with unresolved historical stress that is manifesting as physical symptoms in the body. If we don't have a clear understanding of the true effects of stress on our lives and health, we are in danger of repeating the same cycles of behaviour that are causing our stress over a lifetime.

Health issues such as weight gain and mental health problems cannot be addressed if we don't deal with the root cause of our stress. Living a stress-filled life and being weighed down by the ongoing effects of unresolved historical stress is not a fun place to be, yet this is the reality for so many people who don't learn the effective tools to help them manage and address their stress.

In this chapter, we are going to cover how stress affects mental and physical health and the impacts of your stress on the people around you. We will also be discussing the tools you can use to manage your stress effectively and will be delving into one of the most powerful stress relievers you will ever find.

Your levels of stress can have a far-reaching impact on other people. This is not about making you feel guilty, but it is important to bring awareness to it because it's a subject that comes up regularly with our clients. If you are living in a state of constant stress, everyone who comes in close contact with you is going to be affected.

Let's take the example of our real-life client, 45-year-old Sally who has a lot on her plate and feels she is juggling multiple balls in the air every single day. She has a job, a husband, kids and the usual responsibilities that all those things entail.

By the time she gets home from her stressful job, she is wound up like a rubber band and is frustrated that the kitchen bench is in a mess and her kids haven't emptied the dishwasher and folded the washing like she asked them to that morning. She has to cook dinner in the mess, she remembers she forgot to pick up milk from the supermarket, the kids are arguing and on top of the day she's already had, this is enough to make her cranky and short-tempered. When one of her kids comes to ask her if she's seen his soccer shorts, she snaps. It all comes flying out in a jumbled mess of yelling, swearing and general unpleasantness.

Once she's calmed down, she feels guilty for yelling at her child, apologises and thinks to herself she must really get on top of being grumpy all the time.

If you are stressed and overwhelmed, someone in your near vicinity is likely to be the one on the receiving end of that stress, even if they haven't really done anything wrong. It becomes very easy for other members of the household to blame the person who is under stress, calling them a grump who needs to chill out and then avoiding them as much as possible. What is often overlooked is that what that person needs the most is someone who is willing to shoulder some of the load and offer support.

We see this a lot in a husband/wife or another male/female dynamic, where the woman feels overwhelmed because not only is she working, she is also taking on the bulk of the child minding and household chores. She is constantly tired and worn out and her husband is left wondering what on earth happened to the fun and vibrant woman he married. What he fails to understand is that she is likely feeling burdened by the weight of her responsibilities and she desperately needs help, even if she may not be outwardly asking for it. Often, all it takes to resolve the situation is to involve the husband in a coaching session to help him understand what is happening to his wife on a physical and mental level because of the stress she is under.

Sympathetic and Parasympathetic Dominance

The reason the type of stress we are dealing with today is different from that of our ancestors is because the stress we have today is constant and unrelenting, leading to excessive adrenaline in the body.

We have an important system in the body called the Autonomous Nervous System (ANS), which is made up of the Sympathetic Nervous System (SNS) and the Parasympathetic Nervous System (PNS). The word 'autonomous' reflects the automatic capacity of the body to regulate the things we don't have to think about such as sweating, digestion and heart rate.

The PNS is also known as 'rest, digest and repair' mode and is activated when the body is calm and relaxed. This system must not be suppressed for long periods of time because it carries out all sorts of essential functions in the body, including hormone production, digestion, reproduction, cellular regeneration, heartbeat, respiration and response to inflammation.

The SNS is the opposite of the PNS and is also known as 'fight or flight' mode. This side of the brain activates when something happens to threaten our survival. Any of the stressful events we mentioned earlier can activate sympathetic dominance. When this happens, the first priority of the body is to keep you alive, so it suppresses the non-essential functions of the body.

A typical fight or flight response will include symptoms such as rapid heart rate, adrenal glands releasing adrenaline and cortisol into the bloodstream, the digestive and reproductive systems being suppressed, the body adopting the correct posture to flee (calf muscles tighten, shoulders round forward, head moves to a forward posture), increased sweating and sharpened senses such as hearing and sight.

Because of our modern demanding lifestyles, we may not be fleeing from wild animals but we can be in a state of sympathetic dominance 24/7. This fight or flight mode is intended to get us out of immediate danger, but the human body cannot cope with being in this state over a prolonged period. It needs to be in balance with the rest, digest and repair mode, otherwise the body gets fatigued and certain functions in the body grind to a halt. This is where serious health conditions start to arise.

Adrenal Stress and Fatigue

When our clients complete the adrenal stress quiz, we get an accurate idea of where they are sitting on the stress spectrum on a physiological level.

Our adrenal glands are small, triangular shaped glands located on top of the kidneys. They have the important job of producing hormones that help regulate metabolism, blood pressure, the immune system and response to stress, among other functions. When stress occurs and the body goes into sympathetic dominance, the adrenal glands respond by producing stress hormones (cortisol and adrenaline) to get us through the crisis. This process uses up cholesterol in the body, which results in other hormones suffering because they are lacking their main ingredient. This is known as adrenal fatigue.

Adrenal fatigue symptoms include but are not limited to: difficulty getting out of bed in the morning, persistent feelings of tiredness even after a good sleep, easily feeling overwhelmed, muscle weakness, salt and sugar cravings, mood changes such as mild depression and impacts on the cardiovascular system.

If adrenal fatigue continues over a long period of time, the adrenals become exhausted because they are unable to recharge and cortisol levels start to drop dramatically. Any type of stress – physical, mental or emotional will always end up in the adrenal glands.

Remember, fight or flight mode should always be balanced by rest, digest and repair mode. If this doesn't happen, our adrenal glands can't recharge and the effects can be very serious.

Stress and Weight Gain

The four main triggers that lead to stress and dysfunctional adrenal glands are processed food, environmental pollutants, the pressures of modern life and poor sleep. The consequences of these triggers is that your 'adrenal fat switch' gets switched on. When that happens, your body shifts into survival mode, where hunger increases, energy decreases and food is stored as fat.

Typical modern-day diets have focused on simply reducing the number of calories we eat. The problem with this theory is that this simply puts your body under stress to try and function with less energy input. When stress increases, your adrenal fat switch eventually turns to the 'on' position, so you end up with an increase in appetite and end up over-eating at the end of the diet, regaining the weight you lost. This is one reason why we focus on more of a lifestyle nutrition plan when coaching clients.

Low carbohydrate intake is not the answer to help regulate your hormones and improve adrenal function. For a start, low carb intake leads to poor sleep and higher cortisol (stress hormone) levels. If your carb intake is too low, your cortisol will rise. It does this because when your body's functions need carbs as a fuel source, cortisol will stimulate the liver to release energy into the blood stream. This rise in cortisol can mean two things; poor sleep and extra fat storage.

Stress and the Gut

When the body responds to stress by going into fight or flight mode, the body must direct all its resources towards basic survival. This suppresses the digestive system and can increase inflammation, leading to leaky gut syndrome. Gut health is not a priority for the body when it is in survival mode. Leaky gut syndrome is usually linked to some type of emotional, mental or physical stress and will most likely accompany other health issues, such as weight gain, eczema or hormonal changes.

The remedy for leaky gut is to identify which foods are causing inflammatory reactions in the body and removing them from the diet. When I first started working with a naturopath many years ago, I was diagnosed with leaky gut. I went through a process of hair testing which identified food and environmental allergens. I was able to remove those foods from my diet, allow the gut to heal and gradually the eczema started to recede and eventually cleared up completely.

Stress and Mental Health

When you are in a state of fight or flight, your body is constantly on the defence because it's preparing for an attack (as from the bear or lion in the jungle). Every cell, muscle and organ is primed for what needs to happen next in order to protect you. The problem is, you're not being attacked, but your brain thinks you are.

It becomes super sensitive to light and noise so you can see and hear the danger. You become overwhelmed and the sensitivity to your surroundings starts to wear you down. You feel anxious and are wondering why you are always feeling on edge, even though nothing dangerous is happening. You start to think there's something wrong with you and this can lead to depression. This cycle continues and life becomes tough.

The link between stress and mental illness cannot be underestimated.

Dealing With Stress

Stress has always been a normal part of the human experience and we simply can't avoid it. Modern science has also shown that emotional and mental stress cannot be separated from physical health; one will always impact the other. The key thing to be aware of is that we don't have to be at the mercy of stress. There are many simple tools that can help you deal with stress effectively and we are going to share some of the best ones with you.

Correct your posture

When a hunched posture reflects our internal state of stress, nerve impulses are unable to flow freely from the brain to the nerves and muscles in the rest of the body. An upright posture indicates to the body that it's safe and does not need to be in fight or flight mode. Methods of correcting posture include the following:

- Stand up straight and imagine there is a straight piece of string running through the length of your body and through the top of your head, which is attached to a hook above. This will automatically pull your chest up and out and tuck in the buttocks, creating an upright stance.

- Set up your work desk ergonomically to ensure you are looking straight ahead at your computer screen, not down at it. Be aware of the natural hunched position that results from working on a laptop and try to sit up as straight as possible.

- Lie vertically on a foam roller, with your head and spine on the roller and your feet on the floor with bent knees. This opens up the ribcage to allow the free flow of oxygen and indicates to your body that it is safe. Do this for at least 15 minutes per day. Even better, pop in some ear buds and listen to a relaxing meditation at the same time. I did this consistently throughout my illness and it was an incredible tool for stress relief.

Identify food sensitivities

Have your hair tested to identify food sensitivities, then remove those foods from your diet for three to six months. This will help to heal the gut because you will be removing the foods that can lead to leaky gut syndrome. If you don't want to get your hair tested, we recommend removing gluten, wheat, dairy and eggs as a priority. Most people are sensitive to these foods, even if they don't think they are. None of these foods promote healthy gut bacteria.

Meditation

Calming down the brain is a stress remedy that is often overlooked. This is a mistake because it's the brain that is ultimately responsible for how our body responds to stress. Before you snap this book shut and think, *"Oh, I can't be bothered with that,"* hear us out!

Meditation can be life-changing when it's done regularly, because it trains the brain to be quiet and the body to relax. There are three main forms of meditation that are particularly effective in dealing with stress; guided imagery, body scans and deep breathing.

128

Assess your lifestyle

All efforts to reduce stress on the body, including the ones above will be useless if there are certain lifestyle factors that are preventing this from happening. Things like unresolved trauma, an abusive relationship or a toxic work environment will continue to force your body into fight or flight mode and you will be unable to recover.

If you want to get on top of your stress levels for good, you must deal with your immediate environment and remove yourself from the root cause of stress.

Stress and Forgiveness

As you read earlier in Steve's story, he fought an internal battle with bitterness and resentment towards a family member for many years. Eventually, he became aware that these feelings were doing nothing more than hurting him and preventing him from moving on with his life. When he made the conscious decision to forgive that person, everything shifted, he released the negative feelings and was able to move forward.

Forgiveness is one of the most powerful tools for releasing stress. Negative emotions towards other people play a massive part in our overall state of health and nothing good can come from clinging to them. Pursuing forgiveness is an act of kindness, not only to the person you are forgiving, but to yourself, because you are allowing more peace into your heart and life.

If you are holding onto negative feelings for a certain person in your life, think about whether you are prepared to keep burdening yourself with these feelings, or if you want to set yourself free and forgive. Sometimes we give our clients a 'letter of forgiveness' template so they can begin the process. You certainly don't have to send the letter, but the simple act of writing it (then maybe burning it) can be enough to set the wheels of forgiveness in motion.

One other thing we must mention is that forgiveness is not a one-time action that is done and then forgotten about. Forgiveness is a daily practice and it may take time to feel like you've overcome those negative feelings. It can be helpful to develop a personal mantra that you can refer to each time those difficult feelings come up.

For example, *"These feelings of resentment are not helping me, and I'm choosing to let them go."*

Like anything, practice makes perfect, so persevere and marvel at how much better life becomes when you let go of that burdensome monkey on your back.

We know that dealing with stress is a lot easier said than done, but it's a crucial part of the health puzzle that needs serious attention if you want to be healthy. This concept might be quite confronting if you feel like you're stuck within a situation you can't change.

As an example, when our client Sarah first came to see us, she was struggling to lose her excess weight and couldn't understand why it was so difficult. After further questioning, she revealed she had a very fractious relationship with a family member after they had a falling out. This was a major source of stress in her life which was literally weighing her down, because the stress hormones in her body meant she was unable to shed body fat.

When we coached her through the importance of addressing the root cause of her stress in order to start losing weight, she reached out to her family member and forgave her. Guess what happened next? She started losing weight. By removing that major source of stress from her life, her body felt safe again and was able to release the excess body fat.

Even if you don't think you're stressed, you might be surprised at what feelings are subconsciously lurking in the background and sabotaging your body's capacity to heal.

Are you unhappy in your job? Are you unhappy in your relationship? Is there someone you need to have an honest conversation with?

Even though these things might not affect your ability to function day-to-day, the negative feelings you may have towards the particular situation are still activating a stress response in the body and therefore diminishing the body's ability to recover.

Whatever the root cause of your stress is, or however difficult it is to overcome, you simply must address it to give your body the best chance to heal.

Start the process of being honest with yourself, identifying the source of stress in your life, then put in place an action plan on how you can start to overcome it. This can be difficult to sort through on your own and sometimes we just need a little bit of help. The best thing you can do in this situation is to reach out to a professional such as a counsellor, life coach or health coach to help you unpack the reasons for your stress and help you deal with them.

We're not saying it will be easy, but it's definitely worth it.

CHAPTER TEN

LAVISH YOUR LIVER

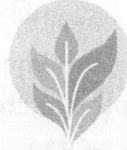

A fundamental part of our coaching programmes is based around healing the liver. That's because it's such a precious organ that has a significant effect on our overall state of health.

Most of us have a sluggish, stagnant or sick liver. We abuse it (either knowingly or unknowingly) with things like caffeine, alcohol, food additives and preservatives, perfumes, hair dyes, air fresheners, scented candles, stress hormones and medications, to name just a few.

Each and every day, our livers are fighting unseen battles for us, doing everything it can to keep harmful toxins from invading our bloodstream and organs.

It's not too farfetched to suggest that the whole world has liver issues. It's estimated that up to 90% of the population has a sick liver and hardly anyone knows it. Most of us don't have a clue about what the liver does and we're certainly not given that information by our doctor, because the link between health and the liver is not fully acknowledged by conventional medicine.

To understand how crucial this organ is to our wellbeing, we must look at the health complications arising from a sick liver, the factors that lead to a sick liver and how to get the liver back to pristine condition if we want to experience great health.

Unless your doctor has investigated the health of your liver, you are probably unaware if it is unhealthy. If, however, you suffer from any health conditions such as autoimmune dysfunction, stubborn body fat, menopause symptoms, chronic pain, mental health issues or sleep problems, it's safe to say you have a sick liver. And it doesn't stop there.

Other issues such as acne, adrenal problems, brain fog, high blood pressure, eczema, insomnia, cysts, methylation problems, sinus infections, urinary tract infections and varicose veins are all a result of a poorly functioning liver.

Because most health conditions stem from an unhappy liver, it's very important to understand what factors contribute to its deterioration and how to initiate the healing process, so your health doesn't continue to worsen. Without this knowledge, it's very unlikely you will be able to resolve your health issues and you certainly won't be able to experience the vibrant health and wellbeing you desire.

In this chapter, we are going to discuss the important role of the liver, what happens when it becomes sick and what you can do to restore it back to full health.

The Role of the Liver

The liver is the unsung hero of the body and controls hundreds, (if not thousands) of crucial functions. It's responsible for important jobs such as storing glucose, glycogen, vitamins and minerals, processing fat and protecting the pancreas, screening and filtering blood and disarming harmful minerals. The liver works hard to keep things balanced in the body, which is a pretty tough ask in this day and age when many of us are feeling overwhelmed and overworked.

The liver is designed to deal with the onslaught of toxins by capturing them, storing them away deep in the liver and then neutralising and detoxifying them to remove them from the body. When the liver becomes sluggish, it is unable to carry out this task and keep you safe, despite its relentless efforts to do so.

Let's take a closer look at some common issues that can stem from an unhappy liver.

Premature Ageing

We're not talking about anti-ageing here, because those words in themselves have connotations of wanting to deny and withhold what is a very natural process. We're talking about ageing prematurely before our time, because who wants that?

There's nothing wrong with wanting to avoid the premature ageing process and it's a very natural part of human nature to resist getting old. Instinctively, we want to hold on to our youth and our health, because the opposite of that is perceived as scary. It doesn't have to be, though.

The desire to hold on to beauty has been a driving force in society forever, ever since Cleopatra bathed in donkey milk and honey to soften and exfoliate her skin. Today, anti-ageing trends are a dime a dozen; everything from supplements, injections, creams, potions and cosmetic surgery to superfoods and diet programmes promise to beat the clock and reverse the ageing process.

Some of those may assist in stalling the ageing process, but most are just fads and gimmicks that generate their producers tons of money while giving us very little in return. When it comes to slowing down the ageing process, the answer is sitting quietly within us and has been fighting our biggest battles since the day we were born. It's the diligent workhorse working behind the scenes to keep our bodies humming while we are oblivious to the fact.

It's the source of our glow, our sparkle and our longevity. The answer is our liver.

If we don't want to age prematurely, we need to give our liver the love and care it deserves. This is the true secret behind staying and looking youthful. We must consciously remove a lot of the junk we are eating, drinking and surrounding ourselves with, because each of these things delivers a king hit to the liver every time we are exposed to them.

Ultimately, we must harness the ability of our liver to keep us young by giving it the goodness it needs.

Fatty Liver Disease

One of the liver's most important functions is to receive blood in huge quantities and then clean, filter and process it. If your blood is thick due to too much saturated fat and too little hydration in the diet, not enough oxygen can reside there. If there's not enough oxygen in the blood reaching the liver, the liver will weaken and become fatty. This is because it is unable to disperse and eliminate fats in the way it is supposed to and it can start to break down and become sluggish. It is unable to draw nutrients from the blood and many of the nutrients end up trapped in fat cells. Toxins also get trapped in the fat cells surrounding the liver and eventually, the liver becomes caked in fat.

Here's a statistic that might shock you:

Worldwide, cases of non-alcoholic fatty liver disease have increased from 391.2 million in 1990 to 882.1 million in 2017. (Ge X, Zheng L, Wang M, *et al*. Prevalence Trends in non-alcoholic fatty liver disease at the global, regional and national levels, 1990-2017)

It's becoming so prevalent that it's very likely you have friends or family members who are either facing premature death or significant health issues at the very least as a result of this disease. This statistic doesn't reflect those who are on the downhill slope with pre-fatty liver disease, either.

These numbers are significant and scary.

Weight Gain

Most people think that weight gain is a result of eating more calories than we burn, or a slow metabolism. The close correlation between a sick liver and weight gain is not really understood or well known. Weight gain is really about the speed at which your liver functions. Liver function has nothing to do with genetics or your body being faulty; it's about what your liver is up against on a daily basis.

We all know that person who can eat all the ice-cream and cake he or she likes and won't put on a single gram. This isn't because that person has a fast metabolism, it's because their liver has not yet been compromised to the point where it's reached its threshold for fat storage.

A compromised liver is not just about the food we eat. There are also several other factors that contribute, which you will see listed under 'Liver Enemies' in this chapter. These include anything that places a burden on the liver, such as chemicals, herbicides, pesticides, plastics, other toxins and excess adrenaline.

In an ideal world, we would all have livers that could deal with toxins, fats and hormones with no problem. In reality, most of us have sick, sluggish and stagnant livers that are breaking down because they are being pushed to their limits every single day.

Mood Disorders

Something that is overlooked within conventional medicine is that mood irregularities can stem from an unhealthy and unhappy liver. Any diagnosis from being emotional to bipolar disorder to Seasonal Affective Disorder (SAD) can have their origins in a sick liver.

When our blood is full of toxins, it leads to a sluggish, pre-fatty or fatty liver. That is, a liver that is over-burdened and struggling with an overload of fat. Add to that those same toxins in the bloodstream that are infiltrating the brain and the curveballs that life throws at us on a regular basis and we have a recipe for grumpiness or sadness, that may then be misdiagnosed as something like SAD.

The liver plays a significant role in our emotional wellbeing but is usually overlooked as a factor in our mental health. To highlight the strong link, think about a time you may have experimented with a 'detox' protocol. When the liver is forced to release its garbage bin of gunk that has accumulated over a long period of time, it can cause an emotional response as the toxins leave. This is why you may feel teary or sad when you are detoxing.

Liver Enemies

There are many 'enemies' our livers have been exposed to since the day we were born. It's important to know what they are if we want to be able to heal the liver and bring it back to life where it can perform at its best. Some of them are already widely known and others you may be surprised by.

If we were to cover every single substance that is damaging to the liver, we would be here forever. So, here's a select few which we think are particularly relevant:

- Petrochemicals: Diesel, gasoline, engine grease and oil, kerosene, exhaust fumes, lighter fluid, gas grills, stoves and ovens, dioxins, paint, lacquer, chemical solvents, solutions and agents, paint thinner, plastics, carpet chemicals.

- Neuro-antagonist Chemicals: Insecticides, pesticides and herbicides, DDT, fungicides, smoke exposure, chlorine, fluoride, chemical fertilisers.

- Food Chemicals: Formaldehyde, preservatives, MSG, aspartame, other artificial sweeteners.

- Foods: Dairy including milk, cheese, yoghurt, eggs, hormones from food, high fat food, alcohol, excessive vinegar use, gluten, caffeine, corn, pork, canola oil, excessive salt use.

- Domestic chemicals: Cologne, perfume, aftershave, hairspray, scented body lotions, sprays, washes, creams, shampoos, gels, air fresheners and mists, aerosol can air fresheners, plug-in air fresheners, hair dye, spray tans, conventional makeup, nail polish and remover, talcum powder, conventional cleaners, conventional laundry powders and fabric softeners, dryer sheets, dry-cleaning chemicals.

- Pharmaceuticals: Anti-depressants, antibiotics, sleeping pills, anti-inflammatories, immunosuppressants, opioids, prescription amphetamines, statins, blood, hormone and thyroid medications, steroids, the pill, alcohol in toiletries, recreational drug use of pharmaceuticals.

- Toxic Heavy Metals: Lead, mercury, aluminium, copper, barium, cadmium, nickel, arsenic.

- Radiation: X-rays, MRIs, CT scans, cell phones, water, food and ongoing atmospheric radiation from nuclear disasters.

This isn't about living in fear or panicking about venturing outdoors. The reality is that we live in a world full of toxins and harmful substances and we can't avoid every single one. What we can do is take ownership over the things we can control and lessen our exposure as much as possible to the things that are harming us.

Adrenaline

Too much adrenaline in the body harms the liver by reducing its ability to perform its intended functions. Adrenaline-based activities such as skydiving, bungee jumping, car racing and free climbing take a huge toll on the liver because the adrenaline is released from the liver in a rush and can create an oversaturation. If you're into doing these activities, you need to make sure you're taking good care of your liver by limiting your exposure to some of the other Liver Enemies.

High Fat Diets

Another area we must pay close attention to when we're talking about liver health is the high-fat diet trend. Over the past several decades, there seems to have been an endless wave of health professionals searching for the 'perfect' diet. We've seen everything from cutting out processed foods to low protein diets to high protein diets to high fat diets and everything in between.

Because western society has an unhealthy obsession with protein (we don't need nearly as much as we're led to believe by the meat and dairy industries), we have ended up eating high animal protein diets. The belief is that animal protein will make us bigger and stronger (it doesn't), but what is overlooked is that high protein diets automatically equate to high fat. Why? Because animal protein is loaded with saturated fat, even the lean cuts.

The high protein (high fat), low carb diets that are on trend at the moment have been repackaged with different names and fancy marketing strategies over the years but are all essentially the same. A few more greens and smoothies have been thrown into the mix, fruit has become the enemy because there's 'too much sugar,' and a few people are noticing some relief from their various niggly symptoms, mainly due to the reduced intake of processed food.

Is the high fat, low-carb diet curing chronic illness though? Definitely not.

Eventually, even the most dedicated and committed people on a high-fat, low carb diet will succumb to the body's needs for natural sugars. The body desperately needs glycogen to keep the brain, liver and other vital organs strong. When the body becomes deprived of glycogen, it becomes desperate and will result in binges on foods like pizza, chips and sugary chocolate bars. Simultaneously, the heart will start to struggle because it's pumping thickened blood (from its high fat content) around the body.

High fat, low-carb diets are not a recipe for a long life. They are a recipe for a shortened life and chronic illness. These types of diets have left a trail of sickness (the Atkins diet) but as time goes on, we forget our mistakes of the past and keep repeating them (the Keto diet).

If you are tempted by a high fat diet because of all the hype and spin and because your friend has lost 5kg by following one, be sure to keep your wits about you. Long term your body will not thank you in the slightest for following this craze.

Healing the Liver

When we appreciate the power of the liver to keep us healthy, our attention turns to how to heal this precious organ. If you know you have an unhealthy and unhappy liver, or if you suspect this might be the case, rest assured that you can bring this workhorse back to life with some tender loving care.

As you've already learned, the liver is burdened by all sorts of harmful foods and things in our environment. Because your liver is working hard every day to protect you, it needs the appropriate fuel to manage its workload. Your liver needs regular meals for sure, but its most important needs are oxygen, water, sugar and mineral salts. If your body is starved of glucose, the liver will slowly starve and cause rapid ageing in the body. Too much fat in the bloodstream will lower oxygen levels and dehydrate the blood.

A key factor in healing the liver is to lower the amount of fat in your diet. Think about all the fats you are consuming at the moment; animal protein, oils, avocados, nuts and seeds and coconut products are all high in saturated fat. Cut the quantity by 25% and bring in more starchy vegetables, greens and fresh fruits instead. Another option is to do some fat-free days to give your liver a turbo-boost in the healing department.

Eating fruit is crucial, because the liver thrives on glucose. Apples are a particularly potent healing food for the liver.

Reducing your intake of alcohol is also important to heal the liver. Alcohol reduces the liver's ability to retain vital vitamins and minerals and slows down its ability to manage its several hundred functions.

Eating regular small meals (grazing) is very helpful in providing the liver with a regular supply of glucose. Eating roughly every two hours will help strengthen the liver and your adrenal glands. You can still have your three main meals per day, just make sure to supplement these with healthy snacks in between.

The following is a list of fantastic healing foods for your liver:

Apples, apricots, artichokes, asparagus, Atlantic sea vegetables, bananas, berries, broccoli, brussels sprouts, carrots, celery, cherries, coconut, coriander, cranberries, cruciferous vegetables (e.g. cauliflower, cabbage) cucumbers, dandelion greens, dates, eggplant, figs, garlic, grapes, hot peppers, kale, kiwifruit, leafy greens, lemons and limes, mangoes, maple syrup, melons, mushrooms, onions and scallions, oranges and tangerines, papaya, parsley, peaches and nectarines, pears, pineapple, pitaya (dragon fruit), pomegranates, potatoes, radishes, raw honey, red cabbage, rocket lettuce, spinach, sprouts and microgreens, sweet potatoes, tomatoes, turmeric, wild blueberries, winter squash, zucchini.

If you're looking at the Liver Enemies list and feel defeated because your job exposes you to petrochemicals or neuro-antagonist chemicals and you have limited control over your environment, the best thing you can do is think about ways in which you can either reduce your exposure to these chemicals (for example, protective clothing, gloves, masks), or at least to the other toxins on the list.

For example, if you work in a horticultural field where you are regularly exposed to things like herbicides and pesticides, try to reduce your exposure to the relevant foods, domestic chemicals and pharmaceuticals as much as possible. Everything we eat, smell or slather on our skin must be processed by the liver, bogging it down and making it stagnant and sick.

If you can limit your exposure to as many of these enemies as possible, you'll be much better off and well on the way to transforming the state of your liver and overall health. We know that plug-in air fresheners smell lovely, but they are one of the most toxic liver offenders you can find. Similarly, while fabric softeners make your towels soft and snuggly, they are actually full of nasty chemicals that your liver has to break down and dispel.

One of the best things you can do right now is to address your nutrition because from here, you will need less reliance on medication to sort out your health issues. Every single pill or tablet you ingest has to be broken down and processed by your liver.

If you're thinking, *"I'm doomed because I've been exposed to too many of these things for too long,"* – don't panic. Your liver is a phenomenal workhorse, remember? It has the most incredible power to heal and rejuvenate if it gets the love and attention it desperately needs. Every day, it's working diligently in the background to keep you safe and well.

If you want to thrive as opposed to just survive, treat your liver with the respect it deserves and you can completely transform your health and life.

It's never too late, but you must start now.

CHAPTER ELEVEN

THE PROOF IS IN THE (HEALTHY) PUDDING

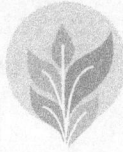

Alex's Story

"From the age of 10, I suffered from a range of symptoms; arthritis in my knees, Irritable Bowel Syndrome (IBS), bladder pain, severe stomach cramps, an inability to stay warm, anxiety, panic attacks, depression, daily headaches, weekly migraines and fatigue, not to mention the complications caused by polycystic ovaries and hormone issues. I don't ever remember having a day where I felt 100%. To be honest, feeling even 50% was like finding the pot of gold at the end of the rainbow.

I have never had the capacity, physically or mentally, to achieve my full potential. As you can imagine, this has compounded greatly into a decline in my mental health, affecting school, work, friendships and other personal relationships, particularly the ability to be there for my son.

I got my first breakthrough at age 23 after 13 years of fighting for help. Finally, I found a doctor willing to listen, research and help. Unfortunately, the medical system let not only him down, but also me. We were going around in circles. I spent weeks off work due to pain or specialist appointments and spent thousands of dollars on appointments, psychotherapy and medications. Let's not forget the immense loss of time spent depressed, lying in bed, or unable to leave my house due to crippling anxiety.

I was very sceptical about Steve and Heidi's programme at first. I had put so much faith in traditional practices, which were supposed to be the most up-to-date, tried and true methods, yet I had hit brick wall after brick wall. How on earth could a 'holistic' pseudoscience possibly help?

I was at my wits end and was so afraid of being brushed aside once again, or my hopes being inflated with grandiose promises of miracles, only to get no further ahead. As unsure as I was, I decided to give their programme a try.

The meal plans were laid out beautifully. They were so easy to follow and integrate into my everyday life. The recipes were delicious, didn't require strange or expensive ingredients and were simple to create, even for a kitchen disaster like myself. I could follow the meals and programme whilst at work, at home with my family and even when out and about on the weekend. Other programmes have felt so difficult to integrate into a normal busy life or require components so expensive that they're unsustainable. One of the diet plans I was placed on by the hospital meant that I was basically restricted to a diet of rice and corn products. No flavour, no variation, no fun.

Now, I have my life back. Energy levels have increased and my ability to face a normal day has now become something I don't even think twice about. My panic attacks and bouts of depression have gone from weekly or daily to barely existent. I have had one migraine since starting this programme and my headaches have reduced to once a month. I have reduced my strong pain medication to only once a week, if that, when I have a flare-up.

My marriage has improved, I am a much better Mum and I am able to spend more time at work. My IBS symptoms have all but disappeared and my arthritic knees are better than ever. I feel like I have a new lease on life. I have my hope back and I am excited to see how far I can go.

I would recommend this programme to anyone and everyone. Most people are told their symptoms are normal, a part of life, part of getting old. Not feeling your best is so widely accepted and this needs to change. If everyone took part in this programme, there would be a dramatic shift in what is considered 'normal'.

Reliance on medication would reduce, mental health would improve and people would have the best possible foundations to get through the hectic and overwhelming lives we lead these days. For anyone who has come to accept their level of pain, weight, mental health, general feelings of mediocrity, who has been told time and time again to 'try this medication' and gotten nowhere, or who has been to multiple specialists or dieticians, this programme is for you. You must stop putting your faith in what we have been brainwashed to see as the 'right' health system and start putting it into something that works.

I can't put into words just how drastically my entire life has changed in the past six months since I've completed the programme. I took part in this programme because I had exhausted myself and all traditional medical options. I had nothing to lose by doing this, and I can't believe it took me 20 years of such hardship, before I finally found Steve and Heidi.

Take the leap, you won't regret it."

Alex Aitken, 31

Tyral's Story

"I had my own business, working long hours in a highly stressful environment with minimal sleep. I thought I had a pretty good diet, but it wasn't really. I was trying to keep active outside of work to reduce some stress as I have always been a keen cyclist and have a general love for the outdoors.

My wife and I had noticed that my health was declining over the past few years, but I had regular check-ups with my doctor and was always told I was fit and healthy. The business was at a point where we could take a decent holiday, so we headed overseas for four weeks and had a great time. I suffer from jetlag really badly, so when I arrived home, I went through the motions of recovering.

Two months later, I felt like I still hadn't recovered. At my worst, I felt like I had severe jetlag, I was tired all the time, had brain fog, a terrible memory and I was having trouble constructing sentences. I started to develop anxiety and had become short-tempered and irritated for no reason.

I eventually went to the doctor for blood tests and they revealed I had a dangerously low red blood cell count and haemoglobin. I was prescribed rounds of Vitamin B12 and another holiday. Over the next five months, I went through a raft of other tests to make sure there was nothing else wrong and I was expecting a significant improvement in health over this time. Although I was feeling better, I was nowhere near where I wanted to be and getting further information from medical professionals was proving fruitless.

With the lack of clarity from the medical profession, I was looking for answers and came across Heidi and Steve's programme. I was a little hesitant at first, but after a phone call my mind was put at rest. I had to make some big changes to my life, including my diet and we had to figure out what was and wasn't working.

I'm not going to lie; there were plenty of two steps forward and ten steps back moments. Often, I was pushing my body too hard or fuelling myself incorrectly. I saw significant changes quite quickly. Brain fog was something I had suffered from for years and this lifted after just a few weeks. Steve and Heidi were great as they listened to me and worked through all the pieces of the puzzle to figure out what was affecting me.

10 months after starting the programme, I completed a five-day mountain bike race and finished mid-pack. I was delighted. I did have to manage my energy and I knew if I pushed too hard one day it would affect me the next. But going from someone who had a hard time getting out of bed and barely being able to string a sentence together, I think I did okay. The programme helped me to make significant steps to recover quickly. It is a long road to recovery and I still have days that aren't so good, but they are few and far between.

Steve and Heidi gave me the tools I needed to heal my body and my brain. I recommend their programme to anyone who isn't feeling at their best and is struggling to get answers from their doctor."

Tyral Roach, 41

Janice's Story

"I had struggled for more than 10 years with stomach issues, including bloating, pain and constipation. I was anxious, not sleeping well and too tired to enjoy life. I was becoming a bit of a social hermit as I would rather stay home and lie flat on the floor to ease the pain. My head was fuzzy and I felt I couldn't

do my job as I struggled to read the computer screen. I had to request a stand-up desk as sitting all day was painful on my gut. My joints ached and I was awake at night with twitchy legs. My issue was not weight gain but the opposite. I am tiny and was lethargic because I wasn't retaining any nutrients from my food.

I had tried absolutely everything from FODMAPs, sleep drops, sleeping pills, probiotics, magnesium, cleansing diets and of course pharmaceutical drugs (Nurofen was my friend to help me sleep!). I had put myself through colonoscopies and many more medical examinations. They were all short-lived remedies and all tests were clear. The doctors said there was nothing wrong with me.

I ended up going to Heidi and Steve in desperation, but to be honest I didn't have much hope and questioned spending the money. My mother-in-law told me about the success of their programme but I was very sceptical as I had already spent a lot of money and time trying so many other options that provided only short-term relief. To be honest, I had decided I just had to live with my problems.

The programme was amazing and the coaching process was very calm, supportive, not pushy and I felt really listened to. I absolutely loved the meals as they were quick, easy and very nutritious.

Learning that carbohydrates are my friend was huge as I love my pumpkin, kumara and pasta but had kept away from these things because I was scared they were causing the bloating. The coaching phone calls each week were a major part of my recovery as I didn't feel alone and my husband didn't have to listen to me complain of my ailments anymore.

Now, I have my energy back, plus I have a good night's sleep 85% of the time. Bloating, pain and constipation have gone 90% of the time. I am a lot less anxious and have the clarity to work through anxious moments. I go out more often and take my plant-based dishes to pot-luck nights and no one even notices!

In fact, I have been asked for my recipes often. My joints only ache when I have walked too fast and my twitchy legs are gone (except when I decided I'm just going to deal with twitchy legs for a night and have a few wines and cheese). Basically, I feel so much better and have so much more energy. My whole family has noticed.

I would highly recommend the programme to others like myself who have ongoing health symptoms and feel like they're 'not quite right' and nothing can be fixed. I truly believe living like that makes us more susceptible to severe illness. I had decided so many things disagreed with me that I had few options left to choose from.

It's very affordable when you break it down to a weekly cost and your grocery bill actually decreases because you are buying fresh foods. It couldn't be easier because you are given your meal plans, grocery lists and recipes each week.

I do have my moments when I go off track but it's not the end of the world. I let myself enjoy certain foods then get back on track the next day. On odd occasions, I end up with a bit of pain but nowhere near what I used to get. I will definitely continue on this journey of healthy living."

Janice Allan, 56

CHAPTER TWELVE

YOUR DAZZLING FUTURE AWAITS

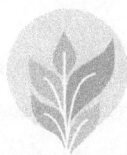

We get very excited when our clients sign up for coaching with us, because we know what they're about to embark on and how their health and lives are about to transform. This part of the book is the equivalent of that, where you get to make a decision that could change the trajectory of your entire life.

In the previous chapters, we have provided you with a ton of information that we base our entire coaching practice on. None of it is crazy, silly, gimmicky stuff, it's just pure and simple awesome information that we use to coach our clients. Did we mention that 95% of the time our clients come to us feeling stuck and disempowered and at the conclusion of our programme, they walk out feeling absolutely fantastic?

That's because this stuff works and we've got stacks and stacks of client testimonials to prove it.

If you're going to make changes in your life, you need to be clear on why you want to make them, otherwise you will stumble at the very first hurdle. Nothing will stick if you aren't sure about the driving force behind your decisions.

In our personal experience and in witnessing that of our clients, each individual has their own unique threshold they must reach before they decide to change. For some, that's a general feeling of being rundown or weighing a few extra kilograms than they feel comfortable with.

For others, it's a cardiac arrest and triple bypass surgery. Whatever it might be for you, it's likely change won't be lasting if you haven't yet reached your threshold of what's acceptable to you because your motivation simply won't be high enough. We're assuming that because you've come this far in the book, you've reached that threshold and are ready to take action.

You also need to become aware of anything that could sabotage your attempts to change.

These things aren't always obvious, but they will slam the door in the face of your best efforts every time if you don't confront them head on. Perhaps the most important factor of all is *how* to implement change and keep it going when things get tough.

> *"We all get scared and want to turn away, but it isn't always strength that makes you stay. Strength is also making the decision to change your destiny."*
>
> (Zoraida Cordova)

There is a very real risk of remaining stuck where you are if you aren't clear on why you want to change, if you are unsure whether your limiting beliefs are holding you back, or if you are unsure how to initiate change and keep momentum. We can't think of anything worse than desperately wanting things to be different but feeling trapped by not knowing how to do it.

We are going to show you how to get clear on your reasons for wanting to take control of your health, the importance of identifying limiting beliefs that may sabotage your efforts and how to activate change in your life that is permanent and lasting.

If you're ready to unleash your personal power and step into the absolute best version of yourself, there's no better time than now!

Goodbye Mediocrity

When it comes to health, we think it's fair to say that most people have mediocre health. They can function okay, get through the day, do what needs to be done, go to sleep and repeat this cycle for the remainder of their living days. We also think it's fair to say that very few people have optimal physical, mental and emotional health. Just look at our overwhelmed medical system as proof of that.

If you have experienced loss of health at any time in your life, you will appreciate how precious it is. Many of us can cruise along relatively well until middle age, taking our health for granted and thinking we're bulletproof, when all of a sudden, whoops! There was a whole raft of health issues festering beneath the surface that have just exploded.

It's a mistake to say to yourself, *"I am ill,"* or *"I have a disability,"* or even, *"My genes are to blame."*

If you think you're sick, you will be sick. Instead, we can train our bodies to overcome limitations and give ourselves confidence to do so in the process.

We want you to know that you don't have to accept mediocre health for the rest of your life. You deserve to experience vibrant health and wellbeing well into your golden years.

 Sadly, we have bought into the myth that aches and pains and niggles are a normal part of ageing and that pills and potions from our doctor will give us some kind of quality of life.

In reality, a huge proportion of our population is on a downward spiral of poor health and depression and are in denial about it, saying they're fine and that it's all just a part of life.

We stand by as observers, passively watching as our bodies age and deteriorate. We accept that we have a certain lifespan laid out for us, without acknowledging how much power we have to influence it. In actual fact, we have the ability to extend our lifespan by maintaining a healthy lifestyle and making daily choices to support that.

It's time to get our heads out of the sand and start learning how to take care of ourselves. We must build strong immune systems and start looking after our livers. We must start making choices that pull us towards life, not death. We need to think about our responsibility to make our lives a blessing not just for ourselves, but for others.

Do You Deserve to Be Happy?

That sounds like a silly question, but one of the key reasons people aren't able to realise their dreams and become the best version of themselves is because deep down they believe they don't deserve it.

Be honest with yourself and ask if this might be the case for you.

If it is, moving towards vibrant health and happiness will be a struggle because your underlying belief will prevent you from taking the necessary steps to get there, even if you aren't consciously aware of it.

Self-sabotage is far more common than you might think.

However, because you are a growth mindset type of person, you will be open-minded and prepared to challenge yourself to overcome limitations. We encourage you to think carefully about any self-sabotaging beliefs that may hold you back.

We all have these beliefs to some degree, but it doesn't mean we need to be ruled by them.

We have seen many clients over the years whose main stumbling block is a deeply held belief that they don't deserve to be happy and therefore, they subconsciously sabotage their weight loss attempts or other health goals every time. They will be incredibly focused and determined, will set some great goals and be well on the way to achieving them, but then their underlying belief systems will take over and sabotage their efforts.

Most of the time people will have no real understanding of why they get to a certain point with their goals, then fall off the wagon. They beat themselves up for being lazy or unmotivated or losing interest, but in fact the real reason is because deep down they don't believe they are good enough to achieve or be happy.

The fear of success can be very real, because it can be uncomfortable to move away from what you've always known into a new and exciting way of being. It can be confronting to think about what people will say or think of you if you change for the better, or how you will feel in your new skin.

If this resonates with you, go easy on yourself. If you know you're doing everything you can to reach your goals but you don't quite get there, it's worth taking a closer look at what limiting beliefs might be sabotaging your behaviour and holding you back. Seeing a reputable life coach can be a great way of getting to the bottom of any self-limiting beliefs and overcoming them.

Mindset should never be underestimated and is so important when it comes to health and wellbeing.

Life by Design

Do you have a goal for the rest of your life? Have you designed what it will look like? What do you want to achieve and who do you want to be?

Most of us ignore the inner power we have to live our best life.

We make small plans about what we will do tomorrow, next week, who we should invite to our dinner party and where to go on holiday. Most of us go with the flow without thinking about the big picture.

A fixed mindset type of person is probably content with that and that's perfectly fine. But, you're a growth mindset person! And in that case, not thinking beyond tomorrow or next week is a colossal waste of your one and precious life.

The overall message behind this book is to inspire and empower you to take control of your health and therefore allow you to put your hands back on the steering wheel of your life. In the end though, it's all up to you. You're not reading this book because you're one of those people who are happy with mediocrity. You're reading it because there's something inside you telling you there is more up for grabs. More health. More life. More spark!

You get to choose what happens next.

Only you know the truth of what's going on with your physical, mental and emotional health and only you have the power to make the necessary changes.

There's a really great quote that we would like to share with you. I heard it while listening to an online interview and in fact, it's one of the catalysts that got us writing this book. This quote is for anyone who is feeling stuck, or not sure what they should be doing with their life, or just needing a sense of direction:

"Go and stand beside the bed of your 95-year-old self and ask them what to do next. They will tell you."

(Katrena Friel)

Think about that for a moment.

Imagine talking to yourself when you are 95-years-old, when you are on your deathbed and about to pass on from this life.

What would they tell you to do next? Would they tell you to fret and worry and not fulfil your dreams? Or would they tell you to get over yourself and go for it? Would they tell you to beat yourself up over all your past failures and hold on to bitterness toward that person who hurt you? Or would they tell you to let it go, take the reins of your life and go forward and fulfil your purpose?

What would they tell you to do about your state of health right now? Would they tell your exhausted self to sit on the couch with a packet of potato chips and a glass of wine? Or would they remind you that you that life passes in a flash and that you're in control of your destiny? Go and ask them; they will tell you.

Another variation on this theme is to write your own eulogy. Think about what you want people to say about you when you die.

What kind of legacy do you want to leave for your loved ones? This can be a very powerful motivator to kickstart change because no-one wants their eulogy to say they sat on their backside too much and wasted their incredible potential.

Get Clear on Your 'Why'

When you get really clear on why you want to make changes in your life, you are more likely to follow through and are more easily able to get back on track when your commitment wavers. Your 'why' will be unique to you and probably quite different to your spouse's or best friend's.

Focus on your reasons only and get really clear about your motivations to take control of your health.

Your 'why' might be about wanting to live a long and happy life. It might be to live to see your children and grandchildren (and great grandchildren) grow up. It might be so you are well enough to travel the world as a backpacker in your 60s. It might be so you are able to tick off every item on your bucket list before you leave this earth. Go wild and think about every single thing you want to do or achieve in however many years you have left.

Bucket list items don't need to be out-of-this-world crazy, but they do need to be things that set your soul on fire.

We always ask our clients about their bucket lists because it gets them thinking about all the things they want to do in their life and puts the spotlight back on whether they will ever be able to do them if they remain where they are right now. Sometimes this is enough to spur them into action, because they are terrified that life will pass them by without achieving their dreams.

If you get excited about your 'why,' you will be more driven to get going and make it happen.

You might be struggling to find it, and that's perfectly okay. You don't score extra points for figuring it out in a heartbeat. Sit with it for a while and let it come to you in its own time. Whatever it is and whenever it makes itself apparent, listen to it, grab hold of it, then go get it!

When you start identifying your 'why' and the items on your bucket list, don't forget to think about the consequences if you don't take action.

Are you prepared to live with those consequences if you remain stuck where you are now?

Find Your Purpose

We have also talked about the fact that, when you are able to identify a purpose or reason for what is happening either now or in the past, you are able to shift your mindset from one of negativity and struggle to one of empowerment. Think about where you are and how you got here and try to pinpoint the reasons you may have had to go through certain experiences in your life.

When we are able to find a reason, our perspective starts to change and we start looking for the positives. This then creates momentum and we are able to confront any future challenges in a more positive way. All of life's challenges make us stronger in the end, even though it's tough to see at the time. Then the next challenge comes along and you are more equipped to deal with it because your previous experiences have given you confidence.

Don't let your past burden you with despair or paralyse you from moving forward.

Use it as a driving force to make today and tomorrow better.

We're not talking about denying reality; more about changing perspective. We can ask, *"What meaning does that thing that happened in the past mean for me now?"* or *"How can I use what I learnt from that event to help me make better decisions in the future?"*

Sometimes it's really hard to look for the silver lining in a difficult situation, but it's even harder to focus on only the clouds. That approach just keeps us stuck in our heads, unable to move forward and make positive change.

Challenge yourself to get unstuck and shift your perspective on what challenging situations mean. What are they teaching you? Are they necessary to give you the experience you need? What kind of person can you become as a result? How can you harness your experience to help someone else?

Have a Plan and a Goal

A plan of attack is a great place to start when you have decided to take control of your health. Take some time to map out a path forward. It doesn't have to be crystal clear, but you do have a better chance of success if you figure out how you're going to get to where you want to be.

Write down your goals, then break down each one into easy-to-do chunks. Think about your current daily routines and habits that need to change, then write down what you will replace those with. Think about any hurdles or obstacles that might derail you and how you will overcome them. Get clear on who you can call on when you need help or a kick in the pants, which leads nicely to our next point.

Enlist Support

One of the reasons our coaching programmes are so successful is because we ensure our clients are supported the whole way through. Don't overlook the value of having a professional standing next to you every step of the way. For us, our job is to give you the tools and support you need, but also to keep you accountable. When people know they have someone to check in with every week they are more likely to stay on the straight and narrow.

Any goal requiring focus and commitment will generate a much higher success rate if the individual has a support network around them to help them stay on the right track. There's nothing noble about trying to achieve a goal on your own. Figure out who your support team will be and tell them what you are about to do. Ask them to keep you honest and pick you up when you fall down or veer off centre.

You might be surprised at who your support crew turns out to be. It's not uncommon for our clients to have limited or no support from the people closest to them and this can be a hard pill to swallow. Wives not supported by husbands; husbands not supported by wives; young adults not supported by a parent.

If you suspect you may be in this boat, remember it's not about you. Changes in your habits or behaviour can be threatening to others because these changes may highlight where they are falling short in their own lives, or perhaps they are afraid of losing the person they know now. Don't take it personally, but quietly go about what you need to do. Hopefully once they see the new and vibrant you, they will start taking an interest and become more supportive.

Also, just because getting on top of your health is a priority for you, it won't automatically be the priority for someone close to you. Not everyone has a growth mindset or is interested in making things better. At the end of the day, don't let their tendency to stagnate in life impact on what you want to achieve.

This is your life, and you get to choose what you do with it. What others do or think doesn't really matter.

Enjoy the Process

Of course, it's all about the destination of great health and a happy life, but it's also about the journey. If you think about it as a daily grind or hard slog, then no doubt it will be.

Mindset, remember?

Find enjoyment in the process of getting to your goal, even if it seems overwhelming or insurmountable to begin with. Nothing good comes easy and it will require work and discipline to get to where you want to be, but it's definitely worth it.

Visualise

Visualisation is a super helpful tool to get you in the zone of taking action. Spend 10-15 minutes sitting quietly at a time when you won't be disturbed. Close your eyes and picture yourself in six months or a year's time.

Where are you?

What are you doing?

Who are you with?

What do you look like?

How do you feel?

What are you able to do that you can't do now?

Go deep with this and see what pictures conjure up in your mind. Visualisation is incredibly powerful because it activates your subconscious mind, programmes your brain, activates the law of attraction and builds internal motivation. A vision board in tangible or digital form is also a great tool to help spur you into taking action.

Go back and read this chapter again if you need to and let it really sink in. As you read through, identify any hesitations or stumbling blocks that pop up.

If you don't think you deserve to be healthy and happy, why not? What can you do or who can help you overcome this belief?

What if you haven't given any thought to what you want your future to look like? It's never too late to get started and make a plan. Time is going to pass anyway, so why not structure it in a way that makes your heart sing?

If you are clueless on your 'why,' give yourself the time and space to figure it out.

What if you aren't confident that you can make lasting change or stay committed through the hard times? Find someone who can support you and hold you accountable.

Are you stumbling through life with no idea about your true purpose? Relax. This isn't something you need to discover in an instant and it doesn't need to be anything sensational or grand.

Start questioning your life experiences and see if you can find a deeper reason for why they might have happened. Where can these experiences take you and what skills have they given you?

What if you don't have a plan and have no idea where to start? Find a good chunk of time when you can be alone to figure out what you need to do and how you will do it. Visualise how you want things to be, then plot the steps on how you will get there.

Nobody is born with a natural ability to sail through life and have everything figured out.

We all have different makeups, personalities, past histories, experiences and skills. You are unique and just by being you, you have a one-of-a-kind combination of these things that nobody else has. How can your unique gifts propel you towards a life you dream of?

Whatever you dream of and whoever you want to be, it's all yours for the taking. But first, you need that one thing that can make it all possible.

That thing that will support you, protect you, fight for you and carry you wherever you desire to go.

That thing that will be your greatest and most loyal friend and your most powerful ally.

That thing is your *health*.

Vibrant health is your birth right. You deserve to be well.

AFTERWORD

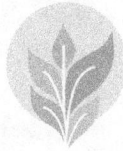

Congratulations for taking the first step towards transforming your health and your life! The information you need to take action is now at your fingertips and we hope you gained immense knowledge and value from this book.

The next step is to harness your new-found motivation because from here, the path forward will begin to take shape. Mapping out a plan needn't be complicated. Go back through each of the five pillars of health and bullet point the things you need to address.

Not everything has to be done at once and the process doesn't have to be rushed. Take your time and remember that small, sustainable changes are more likely to stick in the long term. While the destination of great health and wellbeing is undoubtedly the end goal, enjoy the process and focus on progress, not perfection.

If you are still feeling overwhelmed or need some extra support, please reach out and allow us to walk beside you on the journey.

We have built a successful business on doing exactly that and have worked with thousands of clients who all started exactly where you are now. Often, regular accountability and support makes all the difference between success and remaining stuck.

Above all, remember that your body is designed to thrive and you must trust in its ability to heal. Give yourself the gift of great health and watch as your new way of being unfolds before you.

You have one precious life. Go get it.

ABOUT THE AUTHORS

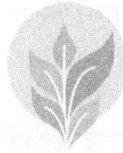

Heidi

Heidi is the youngest of four children and was brought up on an orchard in Katikati, in the Bay of Plenty of New Zealand. After finishing high school, she gained a Bachelor of Arts, majoring in Japanese and International Business Management from the University of Waikato. The allure of travel and living abroad then led to a two-year OE in Japan and the UK.

After working in marketing and local government and seeking a new direction, Heidi completed a Diploma of Holistic Life Coaching through the Life Coach Associates of New Zealand in 2008.

During a health crisis in her late 30s that left her bedridden and disillusioned with conventional medicine, Heidi turned her focus to natural healing and gained a Certificate in Plant-Based Nutrition from Cornell University in the USA. From here, she joined husband Steve in the family business, Jennings Holistic Health Coaching.

Together, their vision is to transform the health and lives of 500,000 people around the world, with a safe and natural approach. Heidi's ultimate goal is to educate and inspire those who are feeling defeated by their health, by showing them how the body can transition from surviving to thriving, given the right tools and support.

Today, Heidi and Steve live in Tauranga, New Zealand, with their daughter Bonnie and son Arie. In her spare time, Heidi loves to dance (Latin American), practice yoga, write for publications on all things health-related and spend time with her family and friends.

Contact Heidi:

W: www.jenningshealthcoach.com
E: heidi@jenningshealthcoach.com
FB: http://Bit.ly/HeidiJenningsPlantBased
http://Bit.ly/JenningsHolisticHealth

Steve

Steve was raised in Katikati, in the Bay of Plenty of New Zealand and is the youngest of five children. Following high school, he moved to Sydney, Australia, where he studied personal training and business management. In 2004, he started his own personal training business and became qualified in Sports Nutrition.

With his professional background in the health industry and being the primary caregiver for his mother and later his wife, Heidi, Steve realised his strengths lay in health coaching.

Jennings Holistic Health Coaching was born and now with thousands of coaching sessions under his belt, Steve finds nothing more rewarding than seeing the health and lives of his clients transform for the better. His goal is to share his story with the world and help lead the health industry into more positive change.

Today, Steve lives with his wife Heidi and two children in Tauranga, New Zealand. In his spare time, he loves sampling craft beer and jamming with his band on the guitar or vocals and is currently producing his first album.

Contact Steve:

W: www.jenningshealthcoach.com
E: steve@jenningshealthcoach.com
FB: http://Bit.ly/JenningsHolisticHealth

Heidi & Steve Jennings

JENNINGS
HOLISTIC HEALTH COACHING

Holistic health coaches Heidi and Steve Jennings are highly sought-after leaders in the health and wellness industry who bring a wealth of knowledge and experience to their field. Their revolutionary blueprint for preventing and reversing illness is second-to-none, with an impressive track record spanning two decades and thousands of satisfied clients.

The Jennings have been featured in national media such as the New Zealand Herald and the Bay of Plenty Times, with Heidi contributing to both domestic and global publications on the subject of health and wellness. In 2021 she was selected as an official honoree for the BRAINZ Magazine Global CREA Awards for her contribution to mental health and leadership.

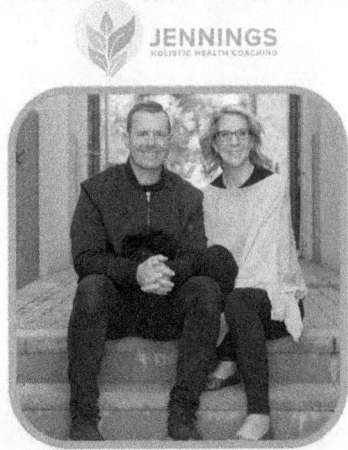

Heidi and Steve's ultimate mission is to spread their message and transform the health and lives of 500,000 around the world. They live with their two children in the Bay of Plenty, New Zealand.

Heidi and Steve can customise their key-note to any audience and time allotment. Their three signature talks are listed below.

Ultimate Blueprint for Optimal Health
- Take control of your health safely and naturally
- Supercharge the healing process
- Achieve life-changing, sustainable results in as little as six weeks

Achieving Optimal Mental Health
- Uncover and address the root cause of stress
- Heal mental health conditions naturally
- How to fuel the body to fuel the brain

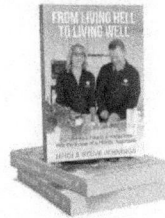

Finding Purpose in Challenging Times
- Why a crisis can be your greatest blessing
- How to turn difficulties into dynamic opportunities
- Why finding purpose and clarity will change your life

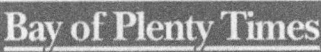

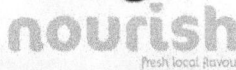

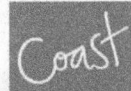

To enquire about engaging Heidi and Steve at your next event, email heidi@jenningshealthcoach.com or phone +64 21 0243 6217 for pricing and availability.

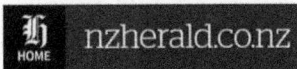

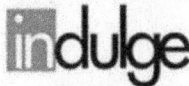

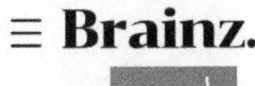

OUR GIFTS TO YOU

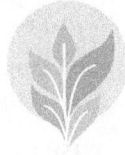

Personalised Coaching Opportunity

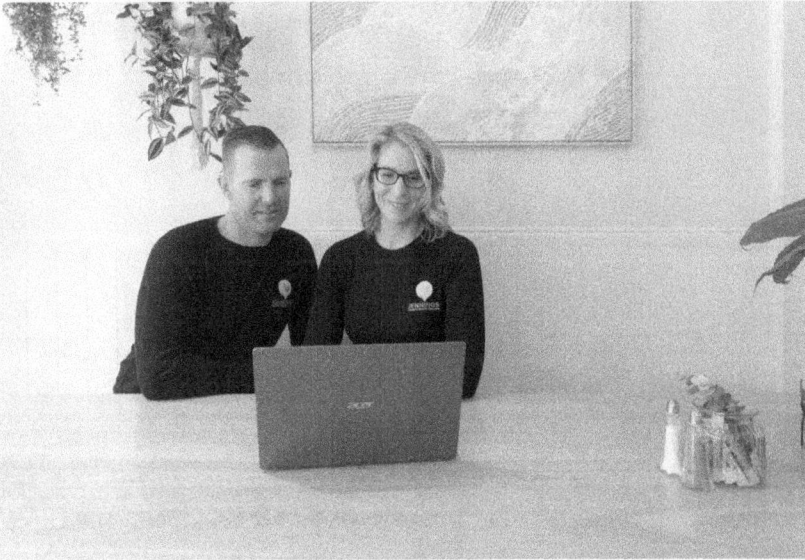

Are you tired of feeling mediocre and like you've lost your spark?

Have you spent time and money going around in circles?

Are you ready to transform your health and unleash your newfound vitality?

Secure a 30 minute Rapid Action session with a proven expert, who will help you map out a personalised path forward and revolutionise your health and wellbeing. If you're ready to become the best version of you, this is a fantastic opportunity not to be missed. Quote *'From Living Hell to Living Well'* to receive a 50% discount off your session. Be quick because spaces fill up fast.

Contact Steve: steve@jenningshealthcoach.com

or Heidi: heidi@jenningshealthcoach.com

www.jenningshealthcoach.com

to secure your appointment.

Complimentary Starter Kit

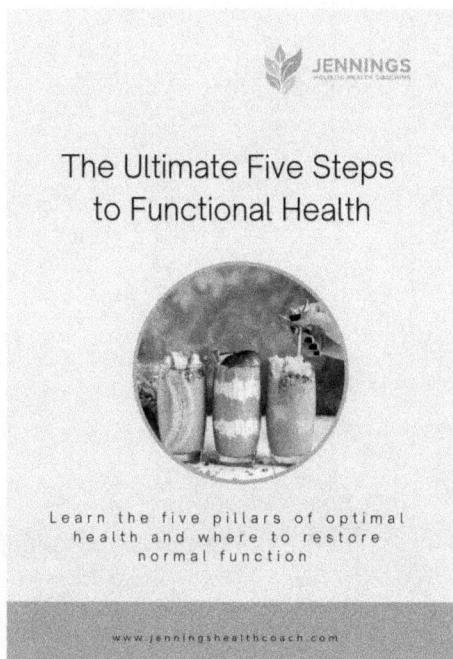

Do you feel stuck or frustrated about your state of health right now?

Are you confused about how to get started on your path to wellness?

Are you ready to take the first steps towards vibrant health?

Download our complimentary e-book, *The Ultimate Five Steps to Functional Health* and identify where you need to take action right now with your health. Get clear on your motivation and reasons for change and take the first steps to completely transform how you feel and show up in the world.

Download your copy at
www.jenningshealthcoach.com/fivefunctionalpillars

HAVE YOU READ *FULL O' BEANS!* YET?

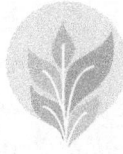

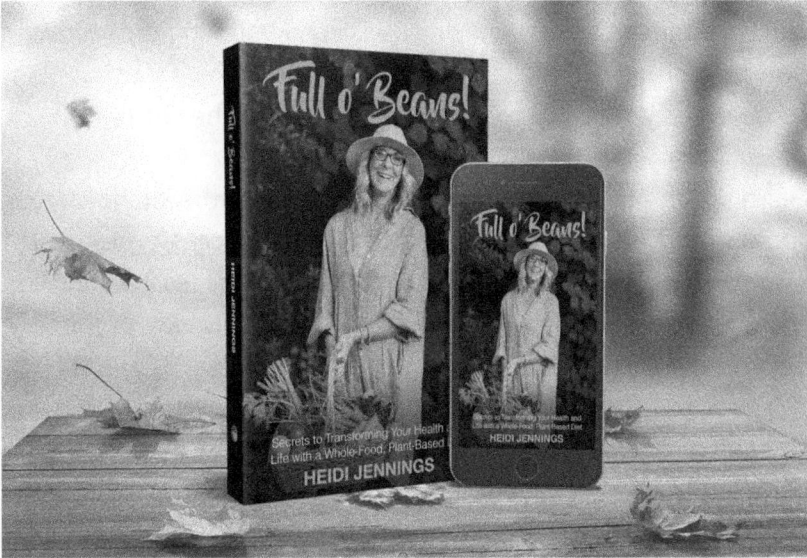

Are you sick and tired of feeling sick and tired? Are you fed up with mediocre or poor health, excessive bloating and gut issues? Are you ready to embrace your full potential, with fabulous wellbeing on your side?

Imagine your own personal wellspring of sublime health, a place to tap into at any time for enduring energy, superb mental clarity and a body that sails smoothly through each day. Think about the feelings of contentment and the kinds of opportunities that a body and mind in perfect harmony would bring.

If this resonates with you, it might be time to look into a plant-based diet.

Following her Amazon #1 bestseller *From Living Hell to Living Well*, holistic health coach Heidi Jennings will take you on an intriguing journey in her latest book, *Full o' Beans!*

From her incredible personal transformation, Heidi shares why our current eating habits are making us sick, how turning to nature can prevent and ultimately reverse disease, and why beautiful plant foods can utterly revamp how you show up in the world.

Learn simple strategies for how to get started in the kitchen, enjoy social situations, set yourself up for optimal success, and so much more. Whether you are struggling with chronic illness, feeling less than your best, or are simply curious about this way of life, this book is a must-read for you.

Get Full o' Beans! and embark on an experience that promises to completely transform your life.

Available for purchase at *www.jenningshealthcoach.com*

ACKNOWLEDGEMENTS

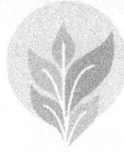

Writing a book is a more challenging and rewarding process than we could have ever imagined. It wouldn't have been possible without Natasa and Stuart Denman and the incredible team at the Ultimate 48 Hour Author: Julie Fisher, Vivienne Mason, Lendy Macario, Nikola Boskovski and Alex Floyd-Douglass. Your guidance, experience and expertise were instrumental in getting the words out of our heads and onto paper.

We are eternally thankful to Heidi's parents and Steve's parents-in-law, Anne and Harry Burggraaf, for your endless support, belief and encouragement. You will never know how grateful we are for everything you do for us.

Thank you to the friends and family members who believed in our story and encouraged us to write it down.

A special thanks to Christine Norton, who generously cast her experienced eyes over our manuscript and offered constructive feedback.

Thank you to Nikki South who captured our cover image perfectly.

To our ex-clients and case studies, Alex Aitken, Tyral Roach and Janice Allan who agreed to tell their stories without hesitation, thank you.

None of this would be possible without our incredible clients. We are so grateful and privileged that you put your trust in us and allow us to walk beside you on your journey towards fantastic health and wellbeing.

And finally, to you, our reader, for choosing to invest in the knowledge we share. We sincerely hope we have given you the tools and inspiration to pursue and obtain the most valuable asset you will ever own; your health.

FURTHER READING

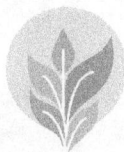

How Not to Die – Dr Michael Greger

The SD Protocol – Dr Wayne Todd

The Autoimmune Fix – Dr Tom O'Bryan

The Adrenal Reset Diet – Alan Christianson, NMD

www.ingramcontent.com/pod-product-compliance
Lightning Source LLC
Chambersburg PA
CBHW032055020426
42335CB00011B/351